Nurse Commitment

Publications by Dr. April L. Jones

Jones, April. "Generational cohort differences among nurses types of organizational commitment in Alabama." 2014. ProQuest (3645920).

Jones, April. "Organisational commitment of nurses: is it dependent on age or education?" *Nurse Management* 21.9 (2015): *29-36.*

Nurse Commitment

How to Retain Professional Staff Nurses
in a Multigenerational Workforce

Nurse Commitment: How to retain professional staff nurses in a multigenerational workforce. Copyright © 2015 by Dr. April L. Jones

Published by Visionary Consulting Services, LLC
www.vcsllc.co
Editor: Kevin Anderson and Associates
Consultant Editor: Bridget Griggs, PhD
Cover Design/Illustrations: Kreashuns Graphics Group
Interior Graphs created by Dr. April L. Jones

ISBN-13: 9781508655671
ISBN-10: 1508655677
BISAC: MED058110: Medical / Nursing / Management & Leadership

Library of Congress Cataloging-in-Publication Data: 2015907330
CreateSpace Independent Publishing Platform,
North Charleston, SC

Printed in the United States of America.

This publication is designed to provide general information about the subject matter covered and does not constitute clinical advice. The author of this work has made every effort to use sources believed to be reliable to the standards generally accepted at the time of publication. This book is sold with the understanding that the author and publisher are not engaged in rendering professional services to the reader.

Knowledge and best practices in this field are constantly evolving. New research and experience broaden our understanding of the subject matter and may require changes in professional practices. Always consult with current research and specific organizational policies and procedures prior to performing any business or clinical procedures. The content is not guaranteed to be correct, complete, or up-to-date.

Practitioners and researchers must always rely on their own experience and knowledge in evaluating and using any methods, charts, table, or others information described in this book. In using such information, they should be mindful of their own safety and the safety of others, including parties from whom they have professional responsibilities. If medical, psychological, legal or any other expert assistance is required, the reader should seek the services of a professional. The information contained in this book is not intended to be a substitute for consulting with an experienced practitioner.

THE INFORMATION PROVIDED IS PROVIDED "AS IS" AND NEITHER THE PUBLISHER, NOR THE AUTHOR, MAKE ANY EXPRESS OR IMPLIED REPRESENTATIONS OR WARRANTIES, INCLUDING WARRANTY OF PERFORMANCE, MERCHANTABILITY, AND FITNESS FOR A PARTICULAR PURPOSE, REGARDING THE INFORMATION. NEITHER THE PUBLISHER NOR THE AUTHOR GUARANTEES THE COMPLETENESS, ACCURACY, OR TIMELINESS OF THE INFORMATION CONTAINED IN THIS BOOK. YOUR USE OF THIS INFORMATION IS AT YOUR OWN RISK.

To the fullest extent of the law, neither the publisher nor the author, contributors, researcher or editors assume any liability for any injury

Dedication

This book is dedicated to my father, the Honorable Lawrence County Commissioner of District 1 Mose Jones, Jr.; my mother, Ella Jones; my sisters, Sharona and Jalisa Jones; my brothers, Shaffer and Christopher Jones; and our Heavenly Father, Jesus Christ. It is because of you that I have accomplished my goal of writing this book. I love you all very much!

Acknowledgments

This book is written in loving memory of my dear grandmother, Ms. Annie L. Jones; my grandfather, Mr. Miller Reed; my cousin, Whitney Jones; my co-worker, Mrs. Melodye Giovanni; community supporters Mrs. Gene Garth, Mrs. Martha Johnson, and "Aunt" Naydean Coffee, RN, for their support and words of encouragement, which will live forever in my heart.

Thanks to my colleagues, Retired Lt Col. Gwendolyn Hill, RN; Ms. Marsha Taylor; Federal Employee/Women members; and Maxwell Air Force Base Protestant Women of the Chapel members for your prayers, support, and motivation to complete this book.

Thank you to my supporters for prayers and motivation, Mary Gilmore-Taite, RN; Ms. Tekeisha Whitt; Miss Jaylynn Harris; evangelist Debra Ward; First Lady Melinda Williams; Mrs. Evelyn Madigan; and, especially my mentor Sandra Harris, PhD, for your coaching, insights on research-writing, motivation, support, and prayers.

Thanks to my sisters-in-law, Veronica Jones, RN and Tamela Jones; my nieces, Alliyah Jones and Tyra Jones; my nephews, Jalynn Jones and Tory Jones; and to all of my relatives for your support as well.

Epigraph

*A*ttention: *healthcare professionals, nurses, nurse managers, human resources professionals and educators!*

Get Their Attention! Maintain Their Retention!

If you have needs to retain your nursing staff and enhance organization effectiveness, but can't due to the current nurse shortage in the US, then here's great news for you.

Discover the Secret to the <u>Retaining</u> Quality Nurses, and <u>Increasing</u> Your Quality of Care, <u>Bolstering</u> Your Employee Relations and <u>Boosting</u> Your Value to Patients!

-Dr. April L. Jones

Table of Contents

Book Reviews

A *brief, targeted book about generational and educational differences in nurses' commitment levels offers health care managers tips on how to maintain staff loyalty. This debut work is the result of the author's six-year Ph.D.–level study of nurse retention in Alabama. In the United States, the nurse-patient ratio is decreasing, with an extreme shortage predicted by 2025. Key to combating this scarcity and the high cost of turnover are the concepts of "organizational commitment" and employee engagement.*

Jones uses Karl Mannheim's theory of generations to discuss the differences among baby boomers, Generation X, and Generation Y (or Millennials) in terms of education, technology usage, and commitment. For instance, baby boomers, who started out in a paper-heavy workplace, struggle to adapt to new technologies; on the other hand, they are dedicated to rising within the ranks of their own organizations. By contrast, Generation X, always searching for higher remuneration, expects little job security ("Members of Generation X are seldom permanent employees because they are always critical of their current position and are frequently on the lookout for better opportunities").

To address frequent sources of dissatisfaction, Jones recommends that managers implement individualized employee development plans. Baby boomers could get more involved mentoring younger nurses, while Generation Xers might enter continuing education programs leading to promotions.

Jones writes in a direct, straightforward style that generally avoids jargon. Managers should appreciate her confident rendering of current circumstances: "everyone seems to be at each other's throat....The Gen Xer is getting really tired of the Boomer constantly looking over his shoulder. He has things under control, why won't she just back off?! "... this work still introduces useful ideas applicable to many staffing situations."

—Kirkus Reviews

Dr. April L. Jones has a Doctor of Philosophy degree in Organizational Psychology which lends her the expertise and ability to analyze business structures and their internal organizations and structures, and her Nurse Commitment addresses a key issue in health management: attracting and retaining nurses.

It applies basic business concepts of team building to the nursing profession with a special eye to managing multi-generational teams, addressing staffing problems not unique to nursing, but to a wider range of business environments.

Six years of research went into the method described here, so this is not just an opinion piece, but a data-supported method that delves into the makeup of multi-generational workplaces and their special challenges.

Chapters consider how employees become committed to their workplaces (or not), how this commitment differs between generations and workplaces, and how employers can foster the kinds of employee dedication that build stronger organizations.

From the emotional challenges of affective commitment to the obligatory responsibility patterns of normative commitment, readers receive an analysis of different degrees of commitment and their patterns of behavior, connections between age and nursing credentials, how managers can use employee development plans with a different eye to implementing better work team models, and how employees can better assess their own progress through worksheets and employer assistance programs.

The result provides a strategic model for a voluntary development program that takes the special strengths and focuses of each different generation into account to build a better overall team.

While nurses and healthcare institutions will be the logical readers of this eye-opening, revealing approach, many a business will want to pursue its infallible logic and attention to building not just explanations and ideals, but an implementable program based on solid research which is heavily footnoted with references and bibliographic materials throughout.

—D. Donovan, Senior Reviewer, The Midwest Book Review

Readers' Comments

It was a pleasure to read Dr. Jones's book on nurse commitment. I found it to be very informative and interesting as she enlightens the reader on the current nursing shortage and offers retention tips based on three different commitment levels as well as generational satisfiers. Nursing leaders should strongly consider Dr. Jones's research when making decisions on how to retain their nurses. Of particular note is the relationship of commitment and engagement to quality patient care or relevance to patient safety.

—Diana Atwell, RN, MSN NEA-BC RN,
Director, Valley Specialty Center
Santa Clara Valley Medical Center/Health and Hospital Systems

This book presents a great comparison of the three different generational cohorts that may be found in the workplace, highlights challenges faced by leaders and explores the various strategic plans needed to increase nurse commitment. The author does an excellent job of showcasing the need for a nurse retention plan based on employee needs and organizational commitment. The reader will come away from this literature with an increased knowledge of other factors that may influence turnover rates and safe nursing environments.

—Christopher B. Robinson, Leadership Development Adjunct
Instructor, Troy University

Generally, the exploration of a multigenerational workforce is a popular and necessary topic, and I'd never appreciated its impact to the nursing field and nurse retention until I read your work! Kudos, Dr. Jones!

—Vanessa Edwards, JD

Aimed at leaders entrusted with maintaining organizational commitment across generations while ensuring retention of the professionals in nursing, a real challenge in today's healthcare businesses....founded on scientific evidence...Dr. April Jones dares leaders to get the best of each generation to get the job done! Yes! Retention is possible if you follow her proposal. Better yet, it can be innovative and self-rewarding for those involved! A must read if you are looking to connect the dots among generational challenges, organizational commitment, and retention.

—Edith Tiencken, GPHR, SHRM-SCP
President and Senior Consultant, SBI International

This book presents a great comparison of the three different generational cohorts that may be found in the workplace, highlights challenges faced by leaders, and explores the various strategic plans needed to increase nurse commitment. The author does an excellent job of showcasing the need for a nurse retention plan based on employee needs and organizational commitment. The reader will come away from this literature with an increased knowledge of other factors that may influence turnover rates and safe nursing environments.

—Clarissa Williams, RN, HCS-D, LHC-COC

The goal should be for all generational cohorts to learn from one another by understanding what each generation can offer to the nursing profession, which in turn would be practical for the internal and external customers as well as the organization to maintaining and retaining all individuals committed to nursing.

—Rosalind P. Gaines, PhD
Specialization in Leadership and Organization Management

Preface

*N*urse Commitment was written after I, Dr. April L. Jones, conducted a six-year study about nurses. Based on the study, I learned that we need to determine and differentiate the types of commitment and understand the generational differences in a workplace. Every person provides a unique value and work ethic. The baby boomer's generation led me to discover that their dedication could assist with retaining nurses from various generational levels because their commitment and dedication could be used as a good example to new nurses.

There is a high turnover of nurses, which is a major problem for health organizations who end up spending more on training and recruiting new nurses. This contributes to a high-risk for patient safety and quality of patient care because there aren't enough nurses to dedicate their time to patients. Due to the shortage of nurses, health organizations have also suffered. Nurses are overworked which can lead to poor motivation and work performance, and less nurse retention.

Through my comprehensive and holistic approach, I discussed the importance of how to work with a team of multi-generational and multicultural nursing cohorts. This book bridges the gap between different generations, providing effective proposals on how to retain nurses who are dedicated and committed to their organization. The book also provides tips about the employee development plan process that will ensure patient safety and quality of care by building organizational stability, organizational effectiveness, and nurse engagement and retention. In this book, managers will learn the essential key on how to communicate and effectively engage with their staff. They will acquire knowledge in observing age differences and analyzing their work preferences so they can understand the value of retaining multi-generational and multicultural nursing cohorts and keep them committed to the organization.

Introduction

Get Their Attention! Maintain Their Retention!

The inability to retain nurses is a major issue for health care organizations, resulting in unnecessary costs, poor work performance, and a loss of patient safety.

Jones's comprehensive and holistic approach focuses on the importance of team building with regard to multigenerational and multicultural nursing cohorts.

Not Just for Nurses!

Jones's methodology, research, and content applies to staffing matrices across the health care environment, and although this book specifically addresses nursing, the principles she presents can be adapted and applied to virtually any industry and profession to increase retention in staffing levels.

Discover Its Unique Strength

Discover the unique strength a cohesive multigenerational cohort brings to your organization's strategic retention plan and philosophy.

Modern multigenerational nursing cohorts come with their own unique challenges, but they can also be leveraged to help retain staff and increase organizational effectiveness.

The Key

"The key is to identify and work with each generation's unique values and work ethic," says Dr. April Jones, who has earned her PhD in Organizational Psychology.

Nurse Commitment is the result of an extensive six-year study, published as an article in the January 2015 issue of the *Journal of Nurse Management* and as a doctoral dissertation in the December 2014 issue of *ProQuest*.

What You Will Discover

- How to **attain new information** to enhance your understanding of generational cohort differences, with work preferences, and get the tools you need to help with a formal employee development plan that will work.
- How to **enhance staff morale** since nurses are afforded opportunities to develop themselves based on their generational cohort work preferences.
- How to **foster respect for generational cohort differences** and work preferences in the workplace, letting nurses know "it's okay to have those desires and it's ok to think outside of the box."
- How to **value diversity among cohorts** in a multigenerational workforce.
- How to **lead more effectively** and manage your staff more efficiently by having a formal process in place.

Understand the UNIT

- <u>U</u>nderstanding generational differences in the workplace is <u>essential</u>.
- <u>N</u>urses are the backbone of the nursing profession and are <u>necessary</u> to ensure patients receive the best quality of care.
- <u>I</u>mplementing a proven professional growth portfolio staff retention and organization effectiveness is <u>paramount</u>.

- Today is the best time to target your team to retain talented nurses because the shortages exist, are all real threats, and the staffing trends aren't improving without <u>action</u>.

Read your copy of *Nurse Commitment* now and let **Visionary Consulting Services, LLC** help you obtain current info to skyrocket your understanding of generational cohort differences with work preferences and get a proven, formal employee development plan.

ONE

The Commitment
Problem: Why It Matters

INTRODUCTION

In US hospitals, the number of nurses per patient is going down. This means much more work for the nurses who are there. As the demand for nurses continues to rise, hospitals are having more and more difficulty ensuring the nurses who remain are committed to their jobs.[1]

The new buzzword floating around hospital administrators is *organizational commitment*. Organizational commitment is defined as "the relative strength of an individual's identification with and involvement in a particular organization."[2].

How invested are employees in their workplace? Are they nine-to-fivers, getting in and getting out, picking up their paychecks and washing their hands of the place? Or do they take pride in where they work? Do they put in that extra effort? Do they want to do what's best for the organization, not just what's easiest for them? Employee commitment to the organization is a critical issue in today's healthcare industry.[3]

---

1 Mary B. Carman-Tobin, "Organizational Commitment among Licensed Practical Nurses: Exploring Associations with Empowerment, Conflict and Trust," PhD dissertation, 2011.

2 R. T. Mowday, R.M. Steers, and L.W. Porter, "The Measurement of Organizational Commitment," *Journal of Vocational Behavior* 14 (1982).

3 G.A. Zangaro, "Organizational Commitment: A Concept Analysis," *Nursing Forum* 36, no. 2 (2001).

Want to know how likely people are to stay with your organization? Check out how committed they are. You can tell, without much difficulty. You can see it in their faces, in the work they do. Ask any nursing administrator; he or she will be able to tell you which ones are still part of the team, and the ones who are looking at the door. That is where commitment comes in. If you can increase your employees' commitment to where they work, you can have a direct impact on the quality of care your patients will receive.

Studies show that different generations have different preferences and needs, which have significant impacts on employees' commitment to organizations.[4] Therefore, a better understanding of their individual expectations and needs will influence healthcare professionals' levels of commitment to their organizations.

THE US HEALTHCARE CRISIS: NURSE SHORTAGE

By 2025, the United States' healthcare system may experience a nursing shortage with losses as extreme as one million nurses.[5] In fact, it is likely that the shortage of registered nurses will worsen until 2030,[6] at which point the southern and western states will suffer an extreme shortage of registered nurses. According to the American Association of College Nursing, by the year 2030, the nursing shortage could contribute to a national healthcare crisis.[7]

---

4 Bryson and White, M.R. Edwards and R. Peccei, "Organizational Identification: Development Testing of a Conceptually Grounded Measure," *European Journal of Personnel Psychology* 16, no. 1 (2007). J.M Twenge and S.M Campbell, "Generational Differences in Psychological Traits and Their Impact On The Workplace," *Journal of Managerial Psychology* 23, no. 8 (2008).

5 P.I. Buerhaus, "Perspective on the Short- and Long-term Outlook for Registered Nurses in the US," *Alabama Nurse* 38, no. 1 (2011); Sephel, Zangaro, "Organizational Commitment"

6 Juraschek et al., "United States Registered Nurse Workforce Report Card and Shortage Forecast," *Amthis erican Journal of Medical Quality* 27, no. 3 (2012).

7 J. Ehrhardt, "Nursing Shortage Still Looms Nursing Schools Warn That Ease In Nurse Shortage Is an Illusion," *Alabama Nurse* 36, no. 3 (2009).

This shortage will result in an increased dependency on licensed practical nurses.[8] Currently, licensed practical nurses within the health-care system execute routine patient care, and they often work at lower wages than registered nurses. However, as the registered nurse shortage worsens, licensed practical nurses may be increasingly called upon to perform tasks usually executed by registered nurses.

This could very likely lead to a decline in quality of patient care, as the average licensed practical nurse has not received the same level of training as a registered nurse,[9] and may be less able to care for the critically injured and ill.

THE CHALLENGE: NURSE ORGANIZATIONAL COMMITMENT

Without organizational commitment, nurses are not engaged in the workplace. This disengagement can directly affect the level of patient care in a hospital.[10] Nurses who are engaged at work do better for their patients. In fact, studies have shown that hospitals with high levels of organizational commitment have lower margins of error than those with low commitment. When nurses are committed, and engaged, everybody wins.

Many different factors go into an employee's level of commitment.[11] The modern workforce is more diverse than ever before. The nursing staff you find at an average hospital is much different than bygone days. Nurses come from a variety of races, genders, ethnicities, and generations. Family of origin, social associations, media, and cultural ties

---

8 Carman-Tobin, "Organizational Commitment."

9 Buerhaus, "Perspective."

10 D. McNeese-Smith and M. Crook, "Nursing values and a Changing Nurse Workforce: Values, Age, and Job Stages," *Journal of Nursing* Administration 33.5 (2003).

11 B. Ashforth, S. Harrison, and K. Corley, "Identification in Organizations: An Examination of Four Fundamental Questions," *Journal of Management* 34, no. 3 (2008). L. Cennamo and D. Gardner, "Generational Differences in Work Values, Outcomes and Person-Organization Values Fit," *Journal of Managerial Psychology* 23, no. 8 (2008). Van Dick

contribute to the different value systems among generations.[12] These generational values are unique within each group.[13] Studies show that different generations have varied preferences and needs, and these distinctions have significant impacts on employee commitment to organizations.[14] It is clear that individual expectations and needs will affect healthcare professionals' levels of commitment to their organizations. It is imperative that researchers investigate the degree to which employees in different generational cohorts differ in their organizational commitment, with an eye to the possible impacts that those differences may have on organizations.

RESEARCH PRINCIPLES
Organizational Commitment Theory

There are several different definitions of organizational commitment. Many researchers understand organizational commitment as the psychological attachment that individuals develop toward an organization.[15] Others define it as the degree to which an individual internalizes an organization's values and goals.[16]

What these definitions have in common is the conception of organizational commitment as one of the main factors in determining things such as employee job performance and satisfaction, personnel turnover, and organizational citizenship behavior. If they want to significantly improve these factors, organizations have got to take a serious interest in their staff's organizational commitment.

---

12 Twenge and Campbell, "Generational Differences in Psychological Traits."

13 Bryson and White, Edwards and Peccei, "Organizational Identification." Twenge and Campbell, "Generational Differences in Psychological Traits."

14 Ibid.

15 Bryson and White, J. Fiorito et al., "Organizational Commitment, Human Resource Practices, and Organizational Characteristics," *Journal of Managerial Issues* 19, no. 2 (2007). P.M. Wright and R.R. Kehoe, "Human Resource Practices and Organizational Commitment A Deeper Examination," *Asia Pacific Journal of Human Resources* 46, no.1 (2007).

16 Somunoglu, Erdem & Erdem

GENERATIONAL THEORY

Karl Mannheim, a Hungarian sociologist writing in the 1920s, is probably the person best known for giving us our concept of generations. His essay, "The Problem with Generations," described how life events shaped people's experience and world views across class, racial, and geographic boundaries.[17] Mannheim believed that, since people who are born in the same period share common life experiences, whole generations tend to share similar thought processes, reactions, and behaviors.[18]

These shared experiences and historical events shape a generation's development of norms, ideals, beliefs, and worldviews.[19] The effect of this stretches across all aspects of life, including work. Applied to nurse's situation, one can say that employment patterns and the particular values of various generations of nurses are based on the social norms and behavioral values developed by each generation.[20]

Generational cycles have historical foundations,[21] and these cycles forecast future movements through the four current types of generations in this country. Each generation has its own specific views about familial roles, traditions, career purpose, work ethics, finance, and life expectancy.[22] We must explore what we know about these generation differences and how it relates to organizational commitment within the workplace today.

---

17 Ibid.

18 Ibid.

19 M.R. Horvath, "Authority, Age, and Era: How to Select Jurors Using Generational Theory," *Verdict* 25, no. 3 (2011).

20 Buerhaus et al., "Impact of the Nurse Shortage on Hospital Patient Care: Comparative Perspectives," *Health* Affairs 26, no. 3 (2007).

21 W. Strauss and N. Howe, *Generations: This History of America's Future, 1584 to 2069* (New York: William Morrow and Company, Inc., 1991).

22 Ibid.

TWO

What We Know About Generations

GENERATIONAL COHORT DIVERSITY IN THE WORKPLACE

Today's workplace is composed of employees who represent a range of generational cohorts.[23] In any given hospital, you can find as many as four different generations of nurses working side by side.[24] These four groups are generation Y, also referred to as millennials, generation X, baby boomers, and veterans.[25] However, the Veteran generation is scarce in the workforce, with the majority of nurses being from generation Y, generation X, and baby boomer cohorts. Because of that, this book focuses mainly on generation Y, generation X and the baby boomers. Generation Y is composed of individuals who were born between 1982 and 2003.[26] The individuals in generation X were born between 1961 and 1981.[27] The baby boomers were born between 1943 and 1960.[28] Generation Y makes up 8 percent of the workforce; generation X makes

23 Cennamo and Gardner, "Generational Differences in Work Value." Giancola; Haynes

24 L. Carver and L. Candela, "Attaining Organizational Commitment Across Different Generations of Nurses," *Journal of Nursing Management* 16, no. 8 (2008).

25 Ibid.

26 Ibid.

27 Ibid.

28 Ibid.

up 21 percent; baby boomers make up 47 percent, and the veterans make up 24 percent.[29]

Each generation has experienced unique events that helped form their belief systems, attitudes, and values.[30] Different nurses experienced the civil rights movement, the fall of the Berlin Wall, the rise of MTV and the destruction of the twin towers during their formative years. And those are just a few examples. Massive cultural shifts have occurred on both a national and global level that have had profound effects on how we view the world. It is inevitable that people who have experienced such radically different worlds growing up would have equally diverse attitudes toward that world.

One example of the differences in experience would be technology. There was a time when nursing was a paper-heavy business. Nurses feverishly scribbled down notes while attempting to decipher pages of instructions, diagnostics, and so on. Now, your modern nurse uses a computer cart. Entering information is all about drop-down menus and data input. For your average gen Xer, this is a welcome advancement. The baby boomers find the changes discomfiting, but they meet the challenge with varying degrees of success. Many Veterans would insist the old ways were better and the millennials cannot conceive of a world where this wasn't the norm. As technological innovation increases, and it is doing so at an ever more rapid pace, these distinctions become even more apparent.

Different generations are, as a rule, going to view things differently. They can vary widely in their attitudes toward behaviors, thoughts and work preferences. Nurse managers must understand these factors, and how they might affect organizational commitment and individual work styles.

---

29 A. Farag, S. Tullai-McGuinness, and M. Anthony, "Nurses' Perception of Their Manager's Leadership Style and Unit Climate: Are There Generational Differences?" *Journal of Nursing Management* 17, no. 1 (2009).

30 Giancola; C. Patalano, "A Study of the Relationship between Generational Group Identification and Organizational Commitment: Generation X vs. Generation Y," Nova Southeastern University, 2008. Tajfel; Turner.

In order to understand the impact of these views, we need to understand the generations themselves- how they think, how they live and how they view their work.

GENERATION Y

Generation Y is frequently referred to as the millennium generation. At over eighty-one members, they account, [31] for approximately a quarter of the U.S. population. Generation Y was born in the age of the Internet and online search engines.[32] As a result, this generation has always had access to technology that other generations did not have during their formative years. This generation of nurses is technologically advanced. Millennials are able to apply their knowledge for practical and efficient patient care.[33] They tend to be comfortable with and skilled at using a variety of technological tools and social media platforms, [34] including Twitter, texting, Facebook, YouTube, Google, and *Wikipedia* websites.

Millennials prefer to work smarter as opposed to harder or longer, [35] which leads to their being perceived as a highly innovative and efficient generation. Generation Y has established new workplace practices under which employees are paid according to their output as opposed to the previous system of being paid according to working hours.[36] Generation Y nurses tend to be civic minded[37] and bring positive changes to healthcare workplaces with core values. These generation Y nurses tend to be tech-savvy and prioritize work-life balance.[38]

---

31 Rawlins; Induik; Johnson and Chang
32 Haynes
33 Morris and Sherman
34 Keeter; Taylor
35 Haynes
36 Giancola
37 Broom; Carver and Candela, "Attaining Organizational Commitment"; Swenson
38 Ibid.

GENERATION X

Generation X is the smallest of the cohorts at only forty-nine million, and its members account for only 17 percent of the US population. This generation of nurses is known for innovation and creative problem solving. They prefer autonomy in their work and resist micromanagement. They are tech-savvy and skilled at problem solving.[39] They are also far less loyal to any given organization, and change employers more frequently than any other generation.[40] Generation X is the most difficult group to retain within a workplace[41] because members are likely to move and are often looking for major prospects that can motivate them to change jobs. Gen Xers believe strongly in self-reliance. They see themselves as self-directed, self-made, and self-sufficient.[42] [43]To successfully manage a member of this generation, leaders have to be prepared to listen to them rather than to simply issue orders. Generation X has a broader vision of advancing in its work. Members of generation X have a zeal for solving larger problems, influencing the status quo, and collaboratively preparing for their futures.[44] They demand respect and involvement.[45] Generation X nurses may be starting out their nursing careers after venturing into business and experiencing the effects of organizational restructuring, downsizing, and workplace re-engineering.[46]

---

39 Buerhaus et al., "Impact of the Nurse Shortage"; Broom

40 Terjesen et al., "Attracting Generation Y Graduates: Organisational Attributes, Likelihood to Apply and Sex Differences," Career Development International 12, no. 6.

41 Ibid

42 Terjesen et al.

43 Mann

44 M. Wong et al., "Generational Differences in Personality and Motivation: Do they Exist and What are the Implications for the Workplace?" *Journal of Managerial Psychology* 23 (2008).

45 Dries, Nicky, Roland Pepermans, and Evelien De Kerpel., "Exploring Four Generations' Beliefs about Career: Is "Satisfied" the New "Successful"?" Journal of Managerial Psychology 23, no. 8 (2008).

46 Wong et al., "Generational Differences in personality."

Generation Xers are aware that successful institutions cannot guarantee them job security,[47] and they do not expect to establish their careers on long-term employment in a given organization.[48] Members of generation X are seldom permanent employees because they are always critical of their current position and are frequently on the lookout for better opportunities.[49]

BABY BOOMERS

Baby boomers have always prided themselves on rejecting traditional values.[50] They are also noted for being slow to embrace changes in the cultural context. Historian Steve Gillon points out that baby boomers, "almost from the time they were conceived…were dissected, analyzed, and pitched to by modern marketers, who reinforced a sense of generational distinctiveness."[51] The baby boomers have received high levels of attention from the generational scholars.[52] Baby boomers see themselves as members of a unique generation.[53] They grew up during a time when social change was taking place at an alarming rate.[54] They experienced drastic changes in the political arena, [55] as well as in every other aspect of life. In terms of social abilities, the baby boomer generation is highly social and rarely prefers individualism. Therefore, they are noted as being able to adapt well to situations that require teamwork, as well as social gatherings.[56]

---

47 McCrindle and Hooper; R. Alsop, *The Trophy Kids Grow Up: How the Millennial Generation is Shaking Up the Workplace* (San Francisco, CA: Jossey-Bass, 2008).

48 Ronald Alslop, *The Trophy Kids Grow Up*

49 Broadbridge et al., "Experiences, Perceptions and Expectations."

50 Connaway et al., "Millennials and Baby Boomers"; S. Dann, "Branded Generations: Baby Boomers Moving into the Seniors Market." *Journal of Product and Brand Management* 16, no. 6 (2007).

51 Gillon

52 Ibid

53 Dann, "Branded Generations."

54 Connaway et al., "Millennials and Baby Boomers."

55 Oblinger

56 Ibid.

Baby boomers tend to be work-centric, and when motivated, they are hardworking.[57] They are often motivated by position, perks, and prestige.[58] They tend to have high levels of independence, [59] self-confidence and self-reliance. Since the generation grew up in an era of reform, its members have a firm belief that they can change the world.[60] They are also goal oriented, which makes them confident in what they want to achieve. In terms of competitiveness, baby boomers are confident in themselves and their abilities.[61] Their desire to win is supported by their positive attitudes toward success. The baby boomer generation of nurses tends to be concerned with career stagnation and prefer face-to-face communication. As a rule, baby boomers have company loyalty, are competitive, and value discussion and working beyond their requirements.[62]

Interestingly, the one characteristic that all generations share is respect.[63] Giving respect to the views and thoughts of each generation is a quick, easy way to earn respect in return.

Understanding these key characteristics is a vital part of managing the various generations. Each demographic has its own set of values and processes. Managers need to acknowledge and practice the most efficient ways to handle the diverse generations.

THE EFFECTS OF GENERATIONAL COHORT DIVERSITY IN THE WORKPLACE

Having all of these different generations in the workplace poses many challenges, especially for management.[64] Managers have to juggle the varying characteristics and expectations of each generation. For exam-

---

57 Ibid.
58 Littrell et al.
59 Connaway et al., "Millennials and Baby Boomers."
60 Dann, "Branded Generations."
61 Oblinger
62 Buerhaus et al., "Impact of the Nurse Shortage"; Broom
63 Carver and Candela, "Attaining Organizational Commitment."
64 Dries et al.; McGuire et al.; Oblinger

ple, a baby boomer is going to be interested in advancing his or her career, while a Millennial is going to want to see great returns. It can be a daunting task. But, managers have to rise to the challenge if they hope to retain these generations within the workplace. And as shortages begin to creep into the hospitals, retaining their workforce is becoming extremely important.

When managers want to motivate their employees, they need to be acutely aware of all these differences.[65] Generation Xers are much more interested in career choices and tend to be driven by work environments that support professional development.[66] In contrast, generation Yers are much more concerned with financial gains.[67] When generation Yers consider the appropriate workplace for them, they focus on what they gain. Strategies to motivate the generation Y employees include incentives such as rewards, pay increases, and other types of workplace compensation. Due to the generations' different motivational needs, human resources within these organizations will be forced to consider including different motivational strategies.[68]

These differences also make it difficult to create any sense of teamwork.[69] It is a challenge to bring together a team composed of varying age groups due to their different priorities.[70] For instance, Shaw and Fairhurst observed that generation is much more oriented toward joining groups and working with other people.[71] Teamwork is a critical part of improving workplace performance. The task of creating a culture of teamwork becomes much more difficult when managers have to contend

---

65 Haynes, Barry P., "The Impact of Generational Differences on the Workplace," *Journal of Corporate Real Estate* 13.2 (2011)

66 Ibid.

67 Yrle et al.; "Generation X."

68 Shaw and Fairhurst

69 K. Macky, D. Gardner, and S. Forsyth, "Generational Differences at Work: Introduction and Overview," *Journal of Managerial Psychology* 23, no. 8 (2008)

70 Ibid

71 Shaw and Fairhurst

with the varying needs of each generation. If managers are going to do it, they need to start by understanding those varying needs.

One way in which having groups of varying generations can cause an issue is when it comes to change.[72] The varying generations have different ways of handling inevitable changes within the organization[73] and having employees who can efficiently cope with change is important. "Generation X is more resistant than other generations when it comes to accepting change, which can cause issues among the staff. Meanwhile, introducing new technology to the workplace often causes problems for the baby boomers.

Here, human resources has to ensure that every generation of worker is motivated to receive the necessary training to use the new technologies.

Generational differences also come in to play in instances of conflict.[74] Oftentimes, it is difficult to even understand where the conflict is coming from due to the age differences involved. At the same time, different generations have significantly different ways of identifying and dealing with sources of conflict.

For example, you find yourself in a situation where everyone seems to be at each other's throat. The older nurse is looking for direction from higher up, and looking to give direction to the gen Xer who falls below her in the pecking order. The gen Xer is getting really tired of the Boomer constantly looking over his shoulder. He has things under control, why won't she just back off?! Meanwhile, he's also stuck dealing with the Millennial who seems to be looking for some kind of validation every ten minutes. Everybody is annoyed, the whole place is a powder keg, and nothing is getting accomplished. This is the world that many managers walk in to every day. That manager, by the way, has his or her own style of doing things, stemming from his or her own generation's mind-set.

---

72 Dwyer
73 Ibid.
74 Macky et al., "Generational Differences at Work"

Determining how to solve this problem requires the manager's understanding of how each of the players goes about solving problems. The Gen Yer, for example, is going to want to brainstorm solutions in a group setting. The gen Xer is going to want to figure out a solution on his own, and then bring that solution to the meeting. The Boomer will be looking for solutions that have worked in the past. These are three very different approaches. None is inherently more productive than the others, but if the group cannot even solve the problem of how to find a solution, what hope do they have?

[75]Differences in organizational competitiveness are critical when it comes to understanding the impact of different generations in the workplace.[76] If managers are going to maximize the organizational commitment of all their nurses, they must first understand the elements that influence each generation.[77] The first step is investigating the use of tools that accurately and reliably measure organizational commitment. Then understanding the different types of organizational commitment among employees and how it relates to their work preferences in order to retain staff and enhance organizational effectiveness.

75 Yrle et al., "Generation"
76 Haynes, "The Impact of Generational Differences."
77 Hunton and Norman

THREE

How Commitment Differs

TYPES OF ORGANIZATIONAL COMMITMENT

It is difficult to measure organizational commitment from a general perspective. To do it right, you need to be able to categorize the different levels of commitment.[78] Understanding the various types of organizational commitment is vital, as it directly impacts the retention and turnover among the various generations. Organizational commitment can be divided into three categories: affective, continuance, and normative.

AFFECTIVE COMMITMENT

Affective commitment is when you have an emotional connection to an organization.[79] An employee with an affective commitment is going to be a big booster for the organization. He or she is always trying to engage others in group activities, refers to his or her coworkers as "family," and feel a deep, personal stake in what happens to the organization. These employees are usually very productive and remain for many years with the organization, possibly for their entire careers. They are the ones who will come to work no matter what. They also tend to feel a heightened sense of group belonging,

---

78 Bryson and White
79 J.P. Meyer and N.J. Allen, "A Three-Component Conceptualization of Organization Commitment," *Human Resource Management Review* 1, no. 1 (1991).

and they demonstrate more collaborative and helpful behaviors.[80] Affective commitment is positively related to prosocial organizational behaviors.[81] Importantly, demographic variables such as tenure, age, year of employment, job type, and marital status have a significant impact on employees' organizational commitment.

CONTINUANCE COMMITMENT

Continuance commitment is a much more pragmatic sort of commitment. It is significantly more calculating than the affective commitment. Essentially, this employee is weighing the time and effort he or she has put into the organization against considerations like potential loss of wages, expenses associated with finding a new job and loss of benefits. This employee is committed because the organization seems like his or her best bet.

Continuance commitment is always thought of in terms of investments and alternatives. Investments are what employees believe they have invested in a job (time, effort, money, etc.) and do not want to lose if they were to leave.[82] Alternatives refer to the employees' perceptions of what is or is not available in terms of alternative employment opportunities.[83] When an employee feels there is too much at stake to leave a job, he or she may have a heightened sense of continuance commitment and be unwilling to accept the risks associated with leaving the position. Basically, this employee stays out of necessity, whether real or perceived.

Continuance commitment works so long as an employee feels he or she has put in a significant amount of time, and that there are not any better options out in the world.

---

80 Den Hartog, Deanne N., and Frank D. Belschak, "Personal Initiative, Commitment And Affect At Work," Journal of Occupational and Organizational Psychology 80, no. 4 (2007).
81 Ibid.
82 Ibid.
83 Ibid.

NORMATIVE COMMITMENT

An employee who feels a normative commitment toward his or her employer feels a sense of obligation and responsibility to continue with that organization.[84] Normative commitment develops when employees adopt the values and support the missions of their organizations.[85] Normative commitment is rooted in employees' cultural values, social norms, and beliefs in organizational loyalty.

These three types of organizational commitment are correlated with how employees commit to an organization, and in turn affects attitudes and behaviors, which affects retention and organization effectiveness. Commitment can be linked to personal initiative, goal-directed behavior, and a willingness to expand effort toward attaining goals.[86] An individual can, over time, have numerous rationales and mindsets toward his or her type(s) of organization commitment depending on his or her perception of attachment to an object within the workforce.

Figure 3.1 offers a pictorial view of organizational commitment and the attitudes and behaviors associated with each commitment type. The core reactions of each type of commitment are one of the following: cognitive (normative commitment), emotional (affective commitment), or motivational (continuance commitment).

---

84 Meyer and Allen, "A Three-Component Conceptualization."

85 Fields; Ashkan Khalili and Arnifa Asmawi, "Appraising the Impact of Gender Differences on Organizational Commitment: Empirical Evidence from a Private SME in Iran," *IJBM International Journal of Business and Management* 7, no. 4 (2012)

86 Den Hartog et al, "Personal Initiative."

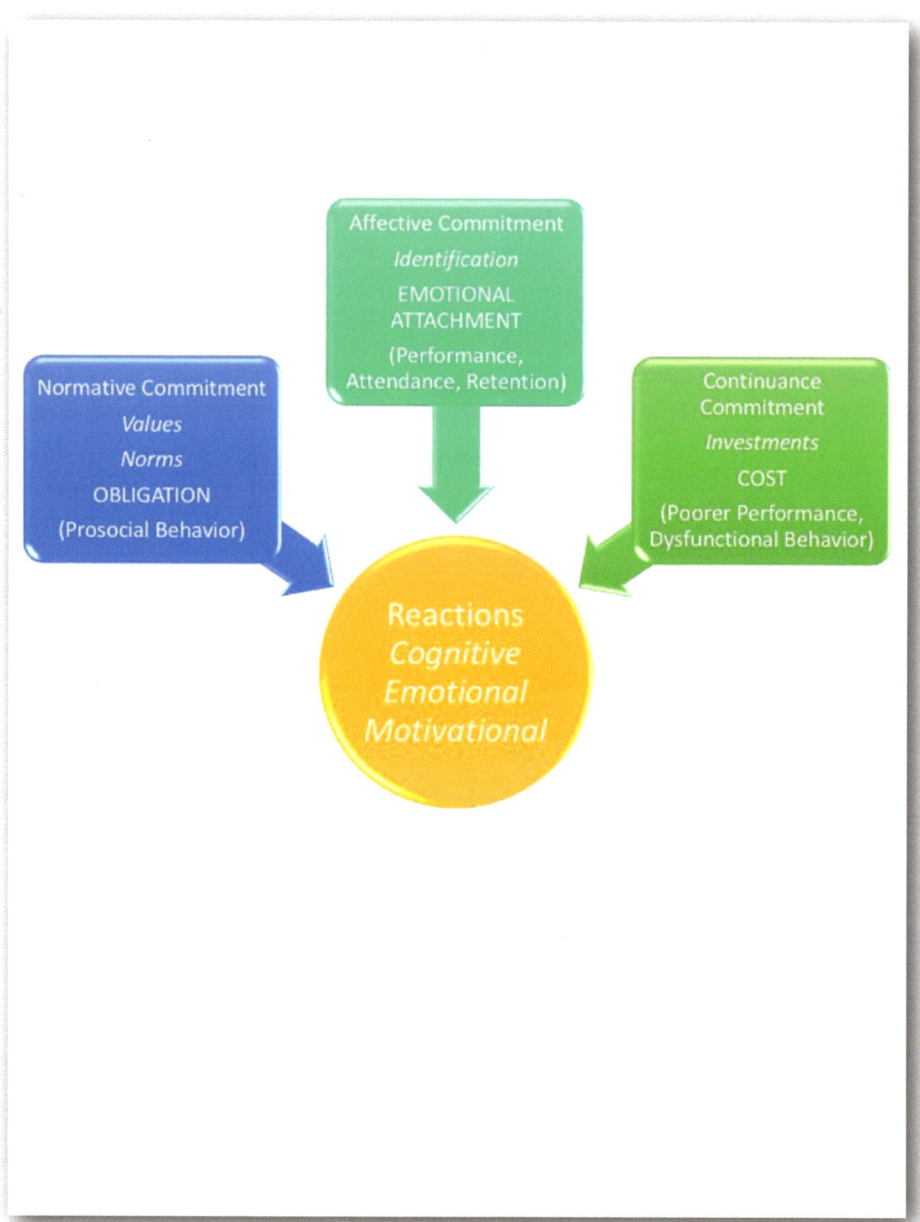

Figure 3.1 Workforce Commitment Reactions Model

FOUR

The State of Commitment Now

THE INTERACTION: AGE AND NURSING CREDENTIALS

My research is focused on nurses employed within the United States. The targeted sample for the study is registered nurses and licensed practical nurses working in the state of Alabama. The participants must have been employed in the state of Alabama in a healthcare setting for at least one consecutive year. My study set out to determine whether three generational cohorts of nurses (generation Y, generation X, and baby boomers) displayed significantly different levels of affective, continuance, and normative commitment. I also investigated whether nurses with various nursing credentials varied in their organizational commitment.

My study revealed some interesting results. Ultimately, generational status is not the key factor in determining levels of commitment in nursing groups. While there are some differences, which I will discuss in more detail soon, a nurse's membership in a specific generation is not the crucial factor in determining his or her commitment to an organization.

The key differences in commitment levels among nursing staff are found when I looked at the different levels of education and certifications among the nursing staff.

The lowest commitment levels are generally found among the LPNs. They are the lowest paid of the nursing staff. At the same time, they possess the lowest level of autonomy. Generally, LPNs are assisting with nursing duties, but they have no ability to make significant decisions regarding patient care. LPNs have the lowest levels of education. An LPN program is a two-year program, usually considered an Associate's Degree. Because their license does not permit it, LPNs cannot sign off on any activity they perform. They are generally used as assistants to the nurses.

A common complaint by LPNs is the lack of authority they have over the decisions they make during their days. LPNs can, at times, be working under nurses who have significantly less practical experience than they, yet they are required by hospital policy to follow the nurses' instructions.

LPNs are most likely to be "paycheck workers." Some LPN's have less interest in contributing significantly to the culture of the hospital. Some are more likely to be seeking a better offer somewhere else. They can also be the hardest to retain on a significant level.

It is important to note that these findings are a general look into the mindsets of the various levels of nursing employees. There are, certainly, many LPNs who work tirelessly to ensure the best possible care for their patients. Most LPNs are very dedicated to what they do, just not necessarily where they work.

These trends are particularly apparent in LPNs of the Baby Boomer and Millennial generations. It makes sense. The Boomers have been working professionally in their career, generally, for quite some time. They tend to go in for prestige and perks. The LPN position has few of either. It is not a glamorous position. It is not a position that garners a great deal of consideration or fanfare among hospital staff. Added to this is the fact that hospital units are changing quickly. Technology is evolving rapidly, becoming a significant part of the day-to-day routine. Boomers, who are slow to embrace such changes, older employees have a tendency to fondly remember the old days, to reflect on how things are changing. "It's not like it used to be," is a common phrase.

Millennials, meanwhile, are searching for positions with levels of compensation that they feel reflect their level of commitment and degree of work. LPN positions are not high paying ones. Millennials see the level of work that comes with being an LPN, and are often frustrated by the lower pay. They often feel that they are undervalued employees. In turn, they value their organization less.

On the other side of the scale, baby boomers with Master's degrees have the highest levels of affective commitment of all subjects surveyed. This makes sense. Boomers are often focused on the level of prestige a position carries with it. Boomers with Master's degrees are more often found in higher positions. Their seniority provides them with a level of authority within the workplace that they value. At the same time, they are more likely to be placed in positions that staff members, as a whole, covet. They have earned the most significant benefits advantages of all the nurses within their unit. Some of them enjoy perks that have been "grandfathered in" from previous policies. They are often found in administrative positions as well.

Ultimately, these trends continue throughout all of my findings. Baby Boomers with Master's degrees tend to have the highest levels of commitment to their organization in all three areas: affective, continuance and normative. On the other end of the spectrum, LPNs tend to have the least. This is particularly true of the Millennial LPNs, who scored lowest in each of the three categories. Boomer LPNs mainly scored low on the affective commitment scale.

These issues are important to bear in mind, because organizational commitment is, as I've said, a key factor in determining employee turnover. As the nursing shortage increases, LPNs will indeed as all professional support staff, become critical pieces of the organizational puzzle. Understanding the mindset of these members of the staff will help reduce employee turnover, increase organizational commitment and improve workplace ratings across the board.

It is particularly important to note that the millennials are the ones scoring lowest across the board in terms of commitment. Arguably, millennials are the future of hospitals. They are just moving into the workforce, and will continue to be a part of it long after their colleagues from previous generations have gone on to retirement.

What all this means is that the group that will be called upon to do the most work for the longest amount of time during any nursing shortage is currently the least committed out of any group to the organizations in which they are employed. This is the workforce of the future, and their participation, and commitment will have a significant impact on how an organization will measure its success for decades to come.

As a factor, generational differences alone do not account for the differing levels of commitment among nursing staffs. The issue, as it turns out, is more complicated than that. In order to fully understand the factors leading to organizational commitment, you also have to account for the level of education staff members have received. The higher their level of education, the higher up the organizational hierarchy they are likely to be found. The lower down that ladder you go, the lower the level of commitment you are likely to find. This is critical knowledge for administrators looking to raise the overall levels of organizational commitment they engender in their employees.

Only when you have taken the time to clearly understand the problem areas, can you begin to consider the potential solutions to those problems for better nurse commitment.

FIVE

Keeping Your Workforce Committed

WHAT THE EXPERTS SAY

A lot of time, effort, and money has been poured into the issue of employee retention. It is an important issue to consider. The costs of employee turnover can be huge. Some estimate that the cost for an organization to replace a specialized employee, and a nurse absolutely qualifies as such, can be as much as 150 percent of that employee's salary. With the threat of a severe nursing shortage, this issue becomes even more of a concern for hospital administrators. They have a very real, vested interest in understanding why employees leave, and what they can do to prevent it.

The research literature suggests strategic plans and reward-based compensation systems for employee retention. These include attractive benefit packages, retention and annual bonuses, student loan repayment, tuition reimbursement, recognition programs, mentor programs, annual rewards, training programs, professional development, wellness programs, and morale activities.

Furthermore, literature specific to nurse retention suggests that nurse managers, healthcare administrators, and human resource managers should empower their professional staff nurses by improving the quality of their work environments with a focus on increasing the nurses' autonomy. Welcoming and supportive social networks must supplement increased practical support. Nurses must be offered the necessary resources and information required to enable efficient and accurate decision making. Additionally, all feedback, including criticism as well as praise, should be based on specific tasks. Another way to improve nurses' quality of work is to pay attention to their opinions and demonstrate concern for their daily work. Finally, one of the most critical support systems for beginning nurses is easy and encouraged access to mentors, which will enable nurses to seek advice while sharing their daily experiences.

Other literature suggests that hospitals implement work-team models to allow the nurses to feel more involved and in control of the decision making process. Self-leadership of this kind often leads to an employee's perception of him or herself as more purposeful, competent, and autonomous. These feelings might result in a rise in the employee's job satisfaction while decreasing the hospital's rate of turnover. In addition to the model of the mentor, social and practical encouragement from the worker's supervisor can lead to a lessening of work-related stress, even as support from peers works to reduce turnover.

My study found that nursing credentials affected the nurses' level of organizational commitment, with licensed practical nurses tending toward the lowest levels of emotional attachment and commitment. Baby boomer registered nurses displayed the highest levels of affective commitment. I found that identifying nurses' generational cohorts and organizational commitments may increase nurse-retention and effectiveness. The conventional strategic plan (strategic nurse-retention plan) may consist of any or all of the following: an organizational development plan; a 360 feedback to assist nurses' with employee development plans (these are explained in detail in the following section); a process designed to improve existing skills, or encourage the acquisition of new skills, and finally, the addition of the organization employee-development plan into an annual performance evaluation that will address the nurses' retention expectations and enhance organizational effectiveness. The expected outcome from the strategic nurse- retention plan is to assist with the organization succession planning to improve nurse commitment to retain professional staff nurses and enhance organization effectiveness.

Table 5.1 illustrates the research findings of my study and the nurses' retention desires. It further illustrates the possibilities of an organizational employee development plan founded on the types of organization commitment among nurses and the nurse-retention expectations from nurses across various generational cohorts.

Genererional Cohorts by Nursing Credentials	Education			AC Commitment Type		CC Commitment Type		NC Commitment Type		Nurses' Retention Desires	Organizational Employee Development Plan
	AS	BSN	MSN	Low	High	Low	High	Low	High		
Baby Boomers (1943-1960) LPN	X			X						Expected rewards: increased pay, benefits, recognition for a job well done, ability to set schedules. Expect social security support, promotion and leadership roles.	Formal Training Cross-Training Continuing Education 360 Feedback Mentoring Coaching
Baby Boomers (1943-1960) RN		X					X		X		
			X		X		X		X		
Generation X (1961-1981) LPN	X			X		X		X		Expect flexible work schedules, education and training opportunities, leadership development, rewards, promotions, increased pay and monetized performance incentives.	Formal Training Cross-Training Continuing Education 360 Feedback Mentoring Coaching
Generation X (1961-1981) RN			X		X						
Generation Y (1982-2003) LPN	X			X						Expect extended orientation program to increase comfort in the workplace, work-life balance, technology, recognition, rewards, full-time employment, training and mentorships.	Formal Training Cross-Training Continuing Education 360 Feedback Mentoring Coaching
Generation Y (1982-2003) RN			X		X						

Table 5.1 Nurse Commitment Table

Studies show that nurses with strong affective commitment and high normative commitment typically are the least motivated to leave and have the highest intent to remain with an organization.[87] Also, nurses with strong affective and normative commitment have stronger work-unit relations. On the other hand, the nurses with continuance commitment profiles show lower performance and more intent to leave the organization. These findings concur with my research findings. The task now is to learn how these results of the types of organizational commitment can help with retention of a multigenerational workforce of nurses.

EMPLOYEE DEVELOPMENT PLANS

Overall, the use of each generation's unique characteristics and types of organizational commitment increases retention rates. The key to retaining a multigenerational professional nursing staff may be the creation of employee development plans (EDPs) for all employees, written in concert with organizations' philosophies and connecting with both the strategic nurse-retention plan and the organization employee development plan. An EDP is a plan completed by an individual for self-development. It normally has a one-year time-frame in which the individual can achieve goals for development; these are reviewed and discussed with a manager to correlate the individual goals with the organization goals.

A useful way of incorporating the EDP is by creating a full, comprehensive program relating to a Professional Growth Portfolio. This portfolio serves as a supplement to a nurse's resume, and includes the development plan as well as growth goals and training desires. This can help to develop the idea of nursing as a lifetime commitment by focusing attention on the future and improvements.

From there, an organization must work to develop a significant buy-in from employees. This is attained by regularly discussing overall strategic goals for the organization. Involving employees in this process provides them with a sense of ownership, as well as the opportunity to make substantive contributions to the planning decisions. Providing employees with an active role in the organizational process can have a significant

---

87 I.R. Gellatly, T.L. Cowden, and G.G. Cummings, "Staff Nurse Commitment, Work Relationships, and Turnover Intentions: A Latent Profile Analysis," *Nursing Research* 63.3 (2014).

effect on how they view their roles. The more they see themselves as collaborators, the more likely they are to be committed to the process.

Employees are then also given specific ideas of how the EDP process can benefit them. This process is designed to strengthen their skill sets and make them better at what they do, just as much as it is to make them better for the organization. The personal benefits become tied with the organizational ones, and their commitment will increase. At the same time, the employee becomes aware that the personal benefits of the new system serves his or her best interests. This is a very effective way of creating greater buy in.

The employee creates the EDP; however, the manager and/or supervisor should ensure that the employee understands how to develop it. Within the EDP are the employee's developmental goals linked to the organization employee development plan, which should effect a return on investment for the nurse and the organization through retention, organizational effectiveness, patient safety and satisfaction, and increase in profit.

One crucial aspect of this plan, which I feel must be mentioned at the outset, is that managers must understand both the process of developing the EDP and the purpose behind it. Before such a program can be successfully implemented, there must be absolute administrative support and understanding. EDPs are not a new concept. They have the potential to be extremely effective in providing employees with understandable, and attainable goals. In order for employees to receive the full benefits of such a system, managers must be seen as being fully supportive of the process.

EDPs are developed to strengthen employees' skills and abilities and to assist with the growth and development for promotion and increased skills. EDP action items come from the organization employee-development plan, which can consist of formal education and training classes or informal trainings, such as cross-training, continuing education, 360-degree feedback, self-help books, coaching, and mentorship. EDPs should focus on no more than three goals per quarter to prevent employees from being overwhelmed. EDPs are to be reviewed quarterly, if possible, to set completion dates and track needs, progress, actions, and actual completion dates, which will lead up to the annual performance evaluation.

Figure 5.1 shows how EDPs flow to affect an organization's overall strategic nurse-retention plan.

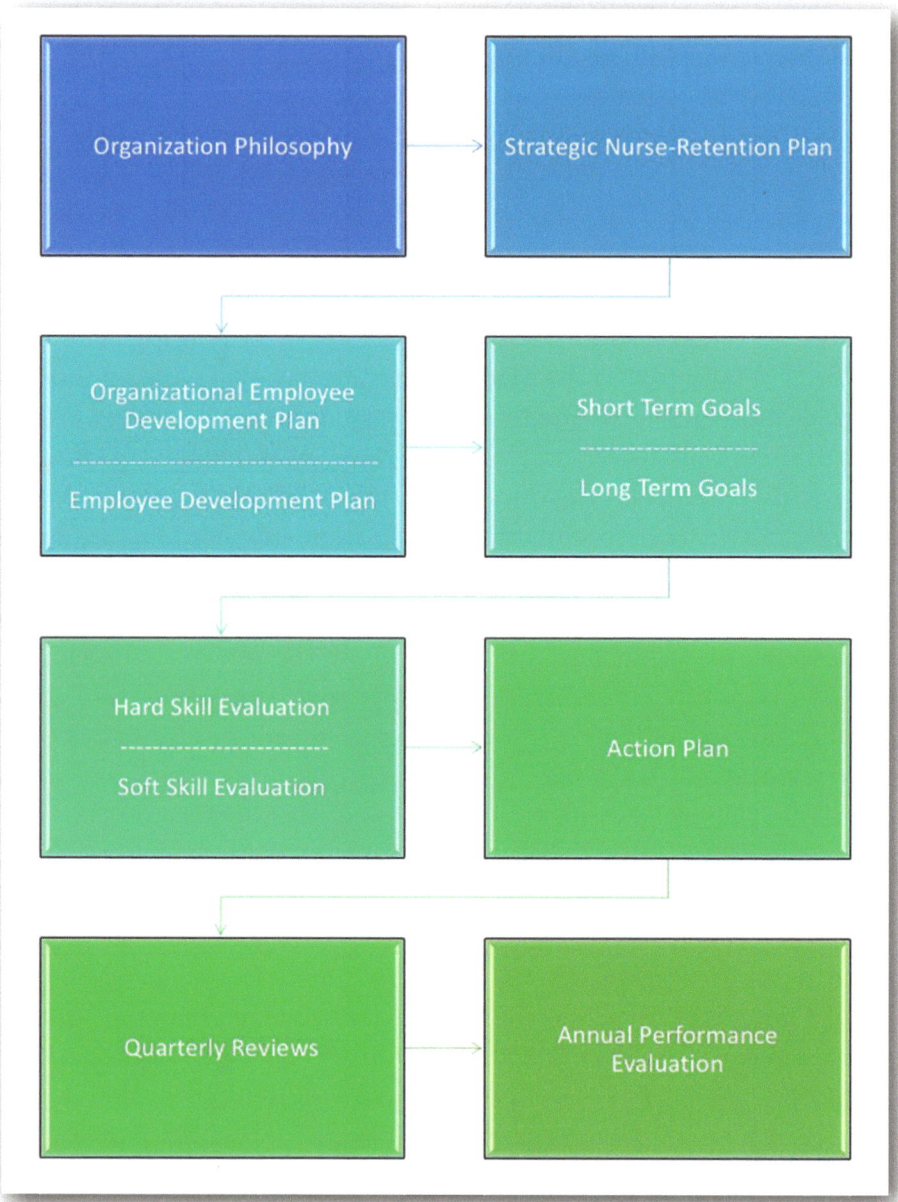

Figure 5.1 Employee-Development Plan Model

This formal EDP may create engaged communication among staff, nurses and managers, as it will devote the proper amount of time to addressing issues and providing opportunities for coaching or mentorship. In Appendix E, The Strength Growth Action Plan (S-GAP) method worksheet is provided as a sample tool to assist with the development of the formal EDP. Quarterly EDP reviews with a manager or supervisor guides the initial education training, and continuing education needs of an employee for growth and development. Annual performance evaluations or 360-degree feedback can assist with promotion, leadership development, and rewards. The plan's outcomes, as shown by these annual performance evaluations, should have review by unit managers, supervisors, and the human resources manager before being compiled for a summary report to the chief executive officer. The chief executive officer will then have a full picture of the organization's retention rates and organizational employee-development needs based on a holistic, strategic approach that positively affects the bottom line. Furthermore, these annual performance evaluations will enable human resource managers to review performance and productivity in order to offer enhanced and versatile benefits packages based on generational cohorts' specific retention needs.

Employees who reach their EDP long- and short-term goals tend to increase production and patient safety and satisfaction, all of which, in turn, increases the organization's revenue and return on investments. These improvements enable an organization to create a diverse benefits package, which could include matching retirement, performance bonuses for appraisals and service, various insurance selections during open enrollment, more full-time nursing slots, and promotion from within by cross-training. Under this system, all entities would work as a whole to make decisions in a process centralized by the EDPs. Unit meeting reports on a quarterly basis would give the group a chance to elevate recognitions and concerns to the human resources manager, where they should be considered for rewards and resolutions.

The most critical aspect of the EDP is that it needs to be an individualized plan. Successful organizations take this aspect of the plan to heart. Employees are provided all the tools necessary, in terms of training and support, to complete a successful, meaningful EDP. Once completed, the EDP becomes a significant benchmark for progress. When the time comes, an employee needs to see the fruits of his or her labor.

Organizations that utilize the EDP model often see significant improvements in employee performance and morale. The goals are met, the employees see that their managers are paying attention, and they feel as though they are actually making progress in their chosen profession. It can send a very clear message that an organization is invested in its employees.

Unfortunately, too many organizations fail to properly take advantage of the EDP system. Many complaints from employees center on improper implementation. Often times, the training or benefits are delayed, or even foregone altogether. This can serve to actually lower employee morale, as it is seen as an overt lack of care.

Figure 5.2 illustrates how a strategic nurse-retention planning model initiates a process with all entities working as a whole to help the organization and employee reach overall long-term goals.

An internal audit of this plan would create a system of checks and balances that would ensure action is taken, and all reports are shared with the managers and floor nurses. The staff that chooses not to develop a full EDP may find some of the plan's components helpful in preparing both a strategic retention plan and an organizational career-development plan.

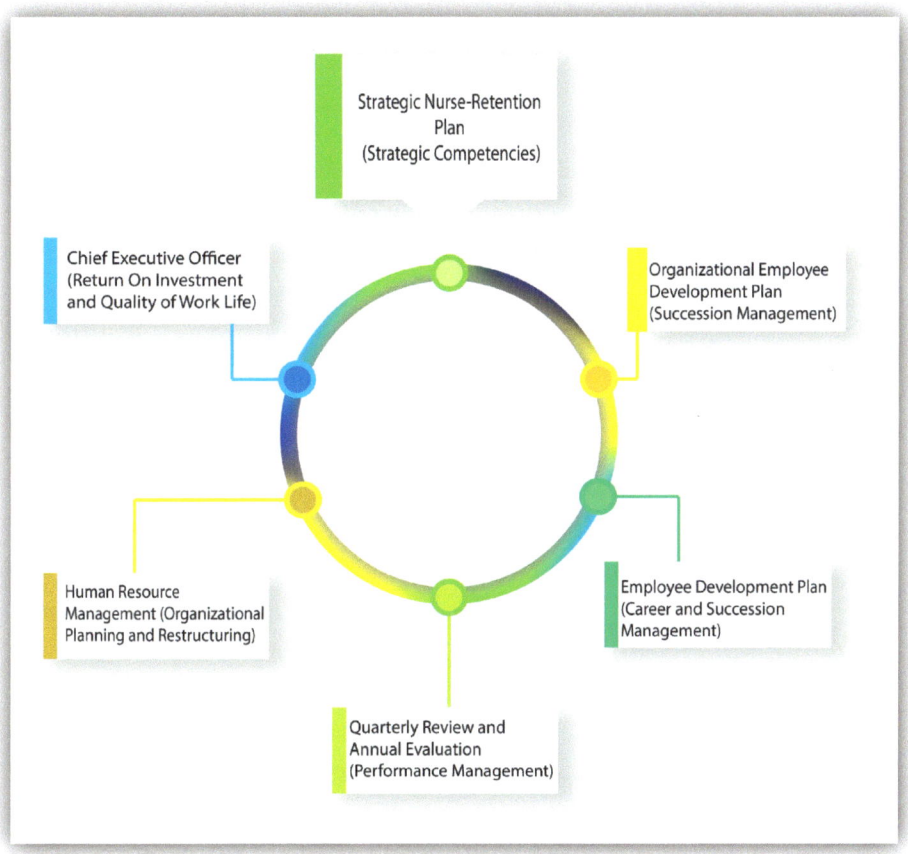

Figure 5.2 Strategic Nurse-Retention Planning Model

WHAT DIFFERENT GENERATIONS WANT
Baby Boomer Retention

Based on my research outcomes discussed in the previous chapter, I suggest a strategic nurse-retention plan based on differing generational needs and organization-commitment types of nurses. The baby boomer registered nurses in this study had the highest overall commitment on all organizational commitment subscales. Therefore, the employment of baby boomer registered nurses appear to be an asset in healthcare settings, as they tend to demonstrate a psychological identification with their workplace.

Baby boomers with senior experience can assist with the retention of younger nurses with less experience, which in turn may increase organizational effectiveness. The baby boomer generational cohort has proven to have the most emotional attachment to the profession, but they also tend to desire more promotion opportunity, autonomy, and efficient communication. Honing in on their particular desires would increase the retention of this talented and experienced generational cohort of nurses that have continued to nurse through many organizational and educational changes. Recognition and use of baby boomers' talents, offering them career advancement opportunities, and making them mentors for novice nurses are logical steps towards increasing retention and effectiveness.[88]

The following suggestions, when implemented by healthcare organizations, would increase the retention rate of baby boomer registered nurses. Options include offering this more senior generation cohort the chance to become nurse coaches or mentors, in addition to making annual pay incentives available based on appraisal performance. The other incentives for baby boomer nurses' might include the following: opening up the possibility of promotion for specialty jobs or management, increasing their involvement with senior leader decisions as a part of a nurse council, and finally, offering set work hours from 6:00 a.m. to 7:00 p.m. The work history of baby boomers has shown that they are

---

88 Buerhaus et al., "Impact of the Nurse Shortage."

especially skilled at working on short notice and following the rules, are often experienced and loyal, and typically appreciate face-to-face communication. Baby boomers' job satisfaction should increase with the use of EDPs focused on utilizing their existing skills as experienced nurses, promotion and recognition, and the development of their leadership skills.

The presence of baby boomers in the workplace may contribute to the other generations adopting the baby boomer's customer service skills and knowledge of how to maintain operations without technology, as well as the preservation of the history of the nursing profession. It may reassert the importance of nurse commitment to quality patient care.

Generation X Retention

In order to retain gen X nurses, employers should ensure they are offering continued education, salaries, communication, and promotion.[89] Generation Xers prefer to work from 8:00 a.m. to 5:00 p.m., and they are eager to learn, autonomous, and skilled with technology. Considering the registered nurse baby boomer's high affective commitment, it is likely that generation Xers, who are mentored or coached by baby boomers, could learn additional information about organization appreciation through the baby boomers' history of nursing through many eras and their customer service skills.

On the other hand, generation X can teach baby-boomer and gen Y nurses additional skills to incorporate technology into their work, the value of continuing education and training, and how to have a work-life balance. Generation X nurses can develop EDPs that incorporate their retention needs, as well as their contributions to the retention of other nurses. The short- and long-term goals of the EDPs are to incentivize buying-in-to the organizational philosophy while also enhancing organizational effectiveness and retention.

---

89 Buerhaus et al., "Impact of the Nurse Shortage."

Generation Y Retention
The article "Impact of the Nurse Shortage" defines generation Y retention needs as mentoring, full-time employment, pay and contingent
rewards.[90]   Generation Y is uniquely tech-savvy. Since its members are
the youngest of the cohorts, the EDP could be very beneficial for generation Y. The experienced registered-nurse baby boomers, working in the
role of mentors or coaches, could be used to retain this generation via
a one-year voluntary development program as a part of the generation
Yers EDP. It could be offered as an option for new nurses as well as for
those with three or fewer years of experience.

The first three months of this voluntary development program can
be spent mentoring in their current clinic or a specialty clinic. The last
nine months can be spent being coached or cross-trained in other specialty clinics and learning new skills, enabling them to achieve promotions and reward opportunities. In return, generation Y can contribute
its technological knowledge and multi-tasking ability to baby boomers
and generation Xers.

Every generation brings with it a unique set of gifts. Whether it is the
millennials' technical savvy, the gen Xers' eagerness to grow or the baby
boomers' experience, everyone has something to contribute to the overall effectiveness of an organization. Like a general, an administrator is
only as effective as his or her troops. Effective leadership requires taking
into account the strengths and weaknesses of the troops, and deploying
them accordingly.

At the same time, each of these generations need to be reached in a
different way, if they are going to be the most effective employees they
can be. Offering a member of generation X a raise, with no apparent
adjustment in position is not going to be the most effective way to ensure
loyalty. Nor is placing a Millennial in a position with more responsibility
but no comparable increase in pay.

---

90 Buerhaus et al., "Impact of the Nurse Shortage."

Organizational Commitment is about more than just salary increases and positions. It is about investing employees with an intrinsic desire to maximize their time within an organization. Each group does it somewhat differently, and each group does it for somewhat different reasons. However, when these groups are given the attention and focus they require, the organization becomes a significantly stronger place for it.

About the Author

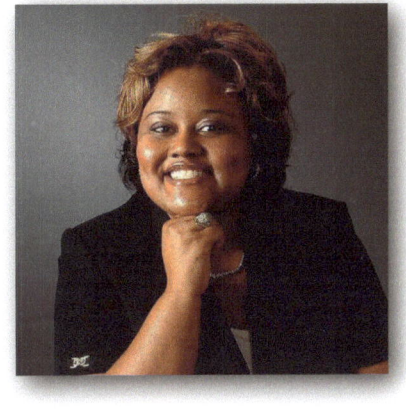

April L. Jones, is a native of Town Creek, Alabama. She currently resides in Montogmery, Alabama. She has sixteen years of experience as a business and social sciences professional. Dr. April Jones is an organizational psychology scientist-practitioner with experience in research, talent management, education and training, human performance management, assessments, public relations, entrepreneurship, strategic planning, leadership development; and, micro and macro social work.

Well known for her ability to successfully engage clients and facilitate dynamic education seminars, Dr. Jones provides subject matter expertise in an array of business consultations.

Dr. Jones's education includes a BA in sociology from Stillman College, a MSW in social work from the University of Alabama, a MS in management from Faulkner University, and a PhD in organizational psychology from Walden University. She is a member of the Alabama State Nurse Association, the American Evaluation Association, the American Psychological Association, Association for Talent Development, the Society of Human Resources Management, and the Society of Industrial and Organizational Psychology, among others. She has presented and/ or been invited to present her research at national and international conferences in Peachtree City, Georgia, Paris, France, Seoul, Korea, Portovoz, Solvenia, Rhodes, Greece, and Brazil.

Appendices

Appendix A: Workforce Commitment Reactions Model

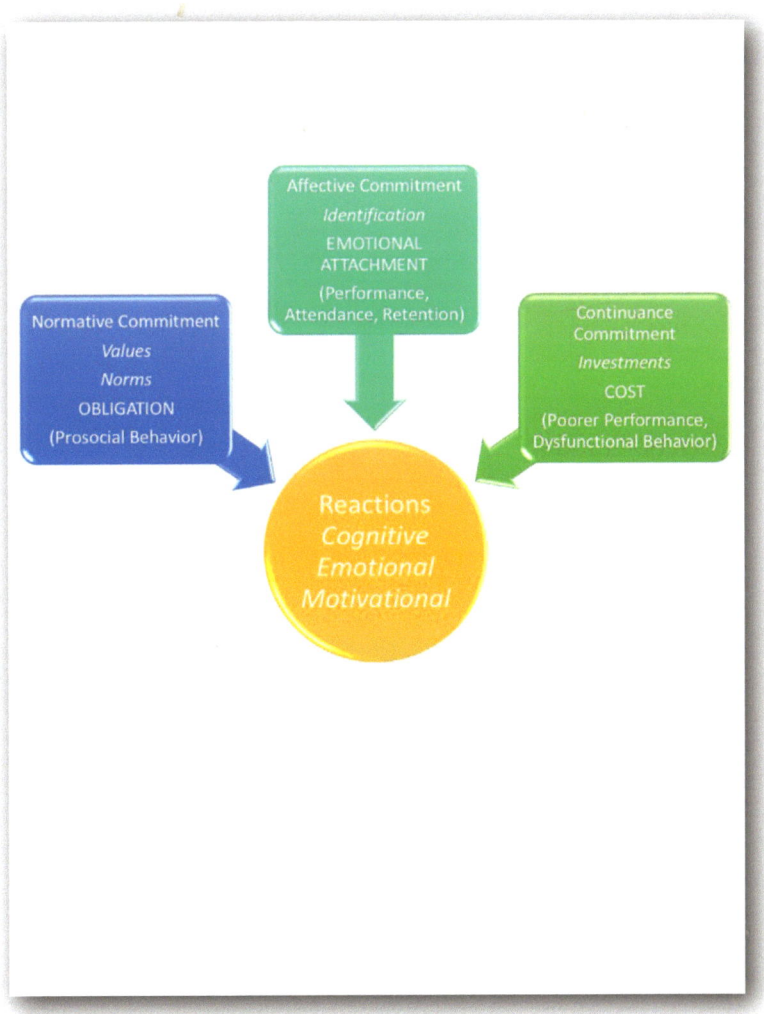

Appendix B: Nurse Commitment Table

Generional Cohorts by Nursing Credentials	Education			AC Commitment Type		CC Commitment Type		NC Commitment Type		Nurses' Retention Desires	Organizational Employee Development Plan
	AS	BSN	MSN	Low	High	Low	High	Low	High		
Baby Boomers (1943-1960) LPN	X			X						Expected rewards: increased pay, benefits, recognition for a job well done, ability to set schedules. Expect social security support, promotion and leadership roles.	Formal Training Cross-Training Continuing Education 360 Feedback Mentoring Coaching
Baby Boomers (1943-1960) RN		X					X		X		
			X		X		X		X		
Generation X (1961-1981) LPN	X			X		X		X		Expect flexible work schedules, education and training opportunities, leadership development, rewards, promotions, increased pay and monetized performance incentives.	Formal Training Cross-Training Continuing Education 360 Feedback Mentoring Coaching
Generation X (1961-1981) RN			X		X						
Generation Y (1982-2003) LPN	X			X						Expect extended orientation program to increase comfort in the workplace, work-life balance, technology, recognition, rewards, full-time employment, training and mentorships.	Formal Training Cross-Training Continuing Education 360 Feedback Mentoring Coaching
Generation Y (1982-2003) RN			X		X						

Appendix C: Employee Development Plan Model

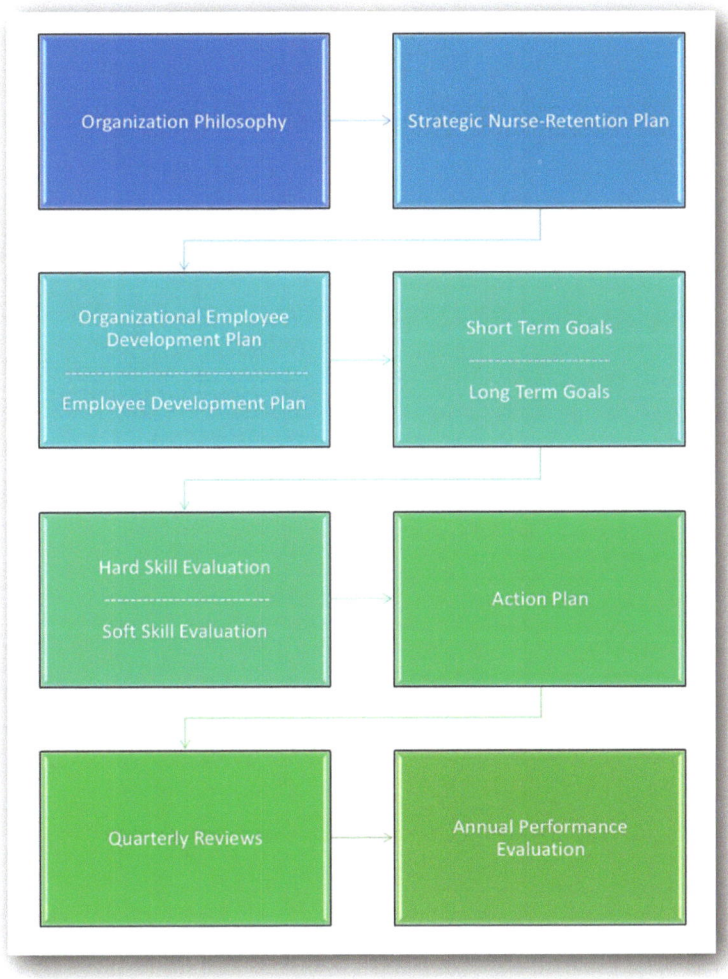

Appendix D: Strategic Nurse-Retention Planning Model

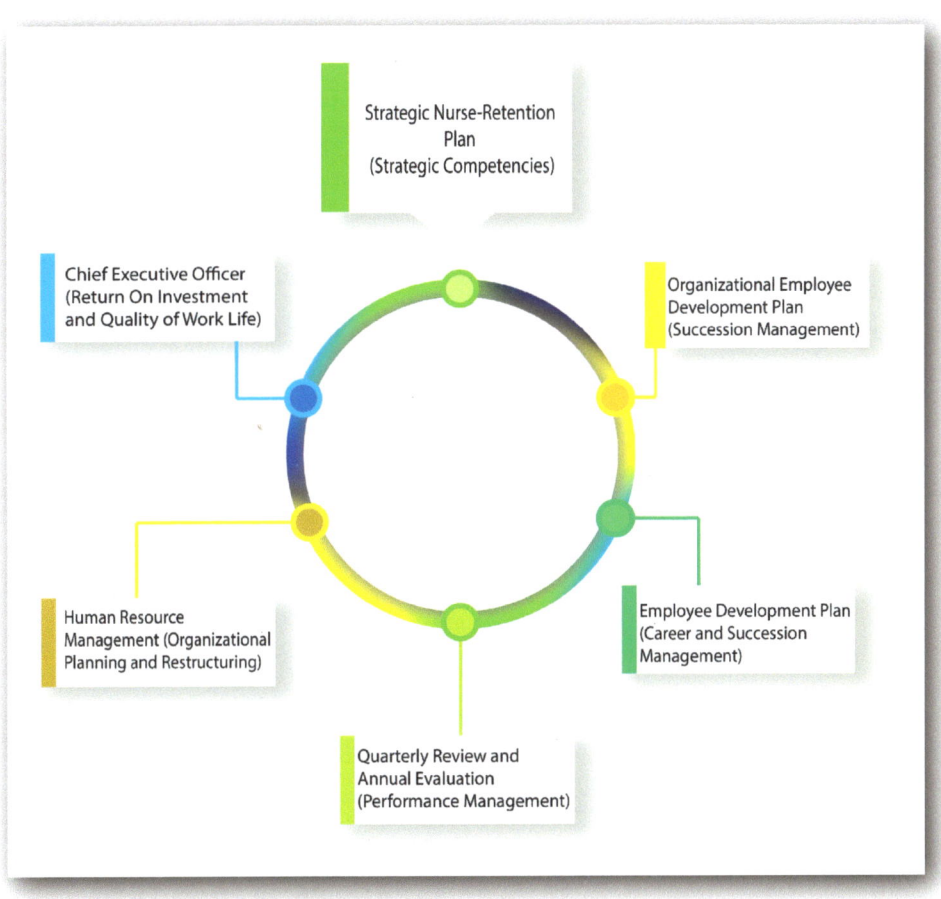

Strategic Nurse-Retention Plan (Strategic Competencies)

Chief Executive Officer (Return On Investment and Quality of Work Life)

Organizational Employee Development Plan (Succession Management)

Human Resource Management (Organizational Planning and Restructuring)

Employee Development Plan (Career and Succession Management)

Quarterly Review and Annual Evaluation (Performance Management)

Appendix E: Strength Growth Action Plan Method

STRENGTH GROWTH ACTION PLAN (S-GAP) METHOD

The **S**trength **G**rowth **A**ction **P**lan (S-GAP) method is an assessment worksheet employees can utilize to assist with the development of their employee development plans to assess and document their quarterly progress toward their annual performance evaluation goals.

Employees should list their top three items in each category to develop their EDPs. The items are subject to change on a quarterly basis depending on mastery of the EDP goals. They should utilize 360 feedback and/or general feedback from managers or supervisors to keep them on target with their goals. The outcomes depend on their performance and the organization's support of their goal(s) achievement.

DIRECTIONS:

Employees should list their top three goals, their strengths, growth needs, the actions based on the Organization Employee Development Plan needed to reach their goals, and the plan to reach these goals for their evaluation outcome(s). The employee should set their completion date(s) when listing goals, the employee should track their progress biweekly (if possible) in preparation for the EDP quarterly meeting with their supervisor or manager. During the quarterly EDP meeting with the supervisor or manager the employee should have their actual completion date(s) listed. They should discuss with their supervisor or managers what helped them meet their goals and/or what prevented them from meeting their goals. The employee should discuss with the supervisor or manager the goals not met for the quarter to discuss solutions that will assist to achieve their goal(s) for the next quarter. Quarterly EDP goal achievements will assist in the success of annual performance evaluation outcomes.

Strength Growth Action Plan (S-GAP) Method Worksheet

Name_____   Date_____

Job title_____

GOALS	STRENGTHS	GROWTH	ACTIONS	EXPECTED COMPLETION DATE	PROGRESS		DATE COMPLETED	PLAN OUTCOMES
					MET	UNMET		

Signature of Employee_____   Manager _____

Appendix F: Skills Assessment Table (SAT)

Some nurses may need assistance with identifying their skills to list their strength and growth needs in the S-GAP method worksheet. The Skill Assessment Table (SAT) is a tool to assist with identifying nursing strength and growth needs that will help with development of the S-GAP worksheet.

DIRECTIONS:

Check the skills that you already have with an X. Then circle the top three growth needs to reach your EDP goals. You may customize your strengths and growth needs by adding to your list using the blank spaces provided in the worksheet.

Skill Assessment Table (SAT)

STRENGTHS	GROWTH NEEDS
Organizational skills	Computer skills
Leadership skills	Confidence
Attention to details	Critical thinking skills
Communication skills	Ethics
Stamina	Commitment to development
-------------------------------	-------------------------------

Appendix G: Tips for Promoting Employee Development Plans

TIPS FOR SUPERVISORS OR MANAGERS

1. Establish rapport with staff to build professional relationships.
2. Value the unique skills of each staff member and utilize them.
3. Promote the organization philosophy to create a shared vision.
4. Acknowledge individual and unit positive outcomes to reiterate the strategic nurse-retention plan by giving kudos to the employee.
5. Develop unit consensus and teamwork.
6. Support growth and development of staff.
7. Discuss with staff how to reinvent and upgrade themselves.
8. Give constructive feedback to enhance performance towards meeting EDP goals.
9. Communicate in detail.
10. Be open to autonomy of staff members.

TIPS FOR NURSES

1. Be energized, open minded, and willing to change.
2. Be accountable for your EDP actions and goals.
3. Develop your leadership skills.
4. Utilize supervisor or manager support as needed.
5. Develop team work skills.
6. Utilize peer review and feedback to reach EDP goals.

7. Set yourself up for success by developing your EDP goals.
8. View learning as an upgrade of your skills.
9. Participate in staff meetings or organization surveys to voice your opinion about employee development desires.
10. View EDPs as an opportunity to re-invent yourself and work towards your individual goals.

TIPS FOR HUMAN RESOURCES PROFESSIONALS

1. Engage with company stakeholders to develop the company strategic plan, the strategic nurse-retention plan, and the organizational employee develop plan.
2. Implement a cost-effective and user friendly high-performance learning and employee management system (LMS) that tracks employee development plans, professional growth and development portfolios, and manages the talent or performance management system.
3. Determine the Strength Weakness Opportunity Threat (SWOT) analysis and expected return on investment (ROI) to your company strategic plan, organizational employee development plan, and expected patient outcomes.
4. Conduct a gap analysis to determine organization training needs to incorporate into the organizational employee development plan services.
5. Create a logical model to evaluate the organizational employee development plan.
6. Conduct a cost analysis to determine whether to outsource organizational development plan services or whether to create an internal program with staff offering services.
7. Onboard leadership by selecting a leader from the leadership team (e.g. unit managers) who is responsible for actively promoting and sponsoring the employee development plan program.

8. Provide training to staff about how to use the LMS and how to create an employee development plan.

9. Organize a plan and schedule of how Human Resources personnel will interact with supervisors, managers, and employees to receive feedback and reports (e.g. surveys, focus groups, manager or supervisor reports) to compile quarterly progress and needs reports that link to the company strategic plans.

10. Incorporate intangible rewards for employees that accomplish their employee development plan goals, such as using gamification, recognition awards or badges, and motivational notes from supervisors or managers in the LMS.

Works Cited

Alsop, Ronald. *The Trophy Kids Grow up How the Millennial Generation Is Shaking up the Workplace.* San Francisco: Jossey-Bass, 2008.

Ashforth, Blake E., Spencer. H. Harrison, and Kevin. G. Corley. "Identification In Organizations: An Examination Of Four Fundamental Questions." *Journal of Management* 34, no. 3 (2008): 325-74.

Broadbridge, Adelina M., Gillian A. Maxwell, and Susan M. Ogden. "Experiences, Perceptions And Expectations Of Retail Employment For generation Y." *Career Development International* 12, no. 6 (2007): 523-44.

Broom, Catherine, and Mary S. Tilbury. "Magnet status: a journey, not a destination." *Journal of nursing care quality* 22, no. 2 (2007): 113-118.

Bryson, Alex, and Michael White. "Organizational commitment: do workplace practices matter?" *CEP Discussion Papers,* (881), (2008) 1-40.

Buerhaus, Peter I. "Perspective on the Short- and Long-term Outlook for Registered Nurses in the US." *Alabama Nurse* 38, no. 1 (2011): 18.

Buerhaus, Peter I., Karen Donelan, Beth T. Ulrich, Linda Norman, Catherine DesRoches, and Robert Dittus. "Impact of the nurse shortage on hospital patient care: Comparative perspectives." *Health Affairs* 26, no. 3 (2007): 853-62. Retrieved from http://search.pro-quest.com/docview/204648125?accountid=14872.

Carman-Tobin, Mary B. "Organizational commitment among licensed practical nurses: Exploring associations with empowerment, conflict, and trust." Master's Thesis, 2011. ProQuest (UMI No. 3494010)

Carver, Lara, and Lori Candela. "Attaining Organizational Commitment Across Different Generations Of Nurses." *Journal of Nursing Management* 16, no. 8 (2008): 984-91.

Cennamo, Lucy, and Diane Gardner. "Generational Differences in Work Values, Outcomes and Person-organisation Values Fit." *Journal of Managerial Psychology* 23, no. 8 (2008): 24-36.

Connaway, Lynn Silipigni, Marie L. Radford, Timothy J. Dickey, Jocelyn De Angelis Williams, and Patrick Confer. "Sense-Making And Synchronicity: Information-Seeking Behaviors Of millennials And baby boomers." *Libri* 58, no. 2 (2008): 123-35.

Dann, Susan. "Branded Generations: Baby Boomers Moving into the Seniors Market." *Journal of Product & Brand Management* 16, no. 6 (2007): 429-31.

Den Hartog, Deanne N., and Frank D. Belschak. "Personal Initiative, Commitment And Affect At Work." *Journal of Occupational and Organizational Psychology* 80, no. 4 (2007): 601-22.

Dries, Nicky, Roland Pepermans, and Evelien De Kerpel. "Exploring Four Generations' Beliefs about Career: Is "satisfied" the New "successful"?" *Journal of Managerial Psychology* 23, no. 8 (2008): 907-28.

Dwyer, Rocky J. "Prepare for the impact of the multigenerational workforce: Transforming Government: People." *Process and Policy*, 3, no. 2 (2009): 101 – 110.

Edwards, Martin R., and Riccardo Peccei. "Perceived Organizational Support, Organizational Identification, and Employee Outcomes." *Journal of Personnel Psychology* 9, no. 1 (2010): 17-26.

Ehrhardt, Jane. "Nursing Shortage Still Looms Nursing Schools Warn That Ease in Nurse Shortage Is an Illusion." *Alabama Nurse* 36, no. 3 (2009): 1-2.

Farag, Amany A., Susan Tullai-Mcguinness, and Mary K. Anthony. "Nurses' Perception Of Their Manager's Leadership Style And Unit Climate: Are There Generational Differences?" *Journal of Nursing Management* 17, no. 1 (2009): 26-34. doi:10.1111/j.1365-2834.2008.00964.x.

Fields, Dail L. Taking Measure of Work: A Guide to Violated Scales for Organizational Research and Diagnosis. Sage Publications: London, 2002.

Fiorito, Jack, Dennis P. Bozeman, Angela Young, and James A. Meurs. "Organizational Commitment, Human Resource Practices, and Organizational Characteristics." *Journal of Managerial Issues* 19, no. 2 (2007): 186-207.

Gellantly, Ian R., Tracy L. Cowden, and Greta G. Cummings. "Staff Nurse Commitment, Work Relationships, and Turnover Intentions." *Nursing Research* 63, no. 3 (2014): 170-81.

Giancola, Frank. The generation gap: more myth than reality. *Human Resource Planning*, 32 (2006): 37

Gillon, Steve. *Boomer Nation: The Largest and Richest Generation Ever, and How It Changed America*, Free Press, 2004.

Haynes, Barry P. "The Impact of Generational Differences on the Workplace." *Journal of Corporate Real Estate* 13, no. 2 (2011): 98-108.

Horvath, Michelle R. "Authority, Age, and Era: How to Select Jurors Using Generational Theory." *Verdict* 25, no. 3 (2011): 1-22.

Hunton, James E., and Carolyn Strand Norman. "The Impact of Alternative Telework Arrangements on Organizational Commitment: Insights from a Longitudinal Field Experiment." *Journal of Information Systems* 24, no. 1 (2010): 67-90. doi:10.2308/jis.2010.24.1.67.

Johnson, Russell E., and Chu-Hsiang Daisy Chang. "Relationships between organizational commitment and its antecedents: Employee self-concept matters." *Journal of Applied Social Psychology* 38, no. 2 (2008): 513-541.

Jones, April. "Organisational Commitment in Nurses: Is It Dependent on Age or Education?" *Nursing Management* 21, no. 9 (2015): 29-36.

Juraschek, Stephen P., Xiaoming Zhang, Vinoth Ranganathan, and Vernon W. Lin. "United States Registered Nurse Workforce Report Card and Shortage Forecast." *American Journal of Medical Quality* 27, no. 3 (2012): 241-49. doi:http://dx.doi.org/10.1177/1062860611416634.

Keeter, Scott, Cliff Zukin, Molly Andolina, and Krista Jenkins. "The civic and political health of the nation: A generational portrait." *Center for information and research on civic learning and engagement (circle)* (2002): 29-36.

Khalili, Ashkan, and Arnifa Asmawi. "Appraising the Impact of Gender Differences on Organizational Commitment: Empirical Evidence from a Private SME in Iran." *IJBM International Journal of Business and Management* 7, no. 4 (2012): 100-10. doi:10.5539/ijbm. v7n5p100.

Littrell, Mary, Yoon Jin Ma and Jaya Halepete "generation X, baby boomers, and Swing: marketing fair trade apparel." *Journal of Fashion Marketing and Management* 9, no. 4, (2005): 407 - 419

Macky, Keith, Diane Gardner, and Stewart Forsyth "Generational Differences at Work: Introduction and Overview." *Journal of Managerial Psychology.* (2008): 238

McCrindle and Hooper; R. Alsop, *The Trophy kids grow up: How the millennial generation is shaking up the workplace* (San Francisco, CA: Jossey-Bass, 2008).

Mann, Sue. "Understanding generation Y." *Professional Manager*, (2008) Retrieved from http://www.managers.org.uk/client_files/ Understanding%20Generation%20Y%20Jul08.pdf

McGuire, David, Rune Todnem By, and Kate Hutchings. "Towards a model of human resource solutions for achieving intergenerational interaction in organizations." *Journal of European Industrial Training*, 31, no. 8 (2007): 592-608.

McNeese-Smith, Donna K., and Mary Crook. "Nursing Values and a Changing Nurse Workforce." *JONA: The Journal of Nursing Administration* 33, no. 5 (2003): 260-70.

Meyer, John P., and Natalie J. Allen. "A Three-component Conceptualization of Organizational Commitment." *Human Resource Management Review* 1, no. 1 (1992): 61-89.

Morris, James H., and J. Daniel Sherman. "Generalizability of an organizational commitment model." *Academy of management Journal* 24, no. 3 (1981): 512-526.

Mowday, Richard T., Richard M. Steers, and Lyman W. Porter. "Organizational Commitment Questionnaire." *Journal of Vocational Behavior* 14 (1982): 224-47.

Oblinger, Diana. "Boomers, Gen-Xers & millennials." *Educause Review*, 38, no. 4 (2003): 36-45

Patalano, Carla. "A study of the relationship between generational group identification and organizational commitment: Generation X vs. Generation Y." Nova Southeastern University, 2008. *ProQuest* (304810041).

Rawlins, Brad R. "Measuring the relationship between organizational transparency and employee trust." (2008).

Shaw, Sue, and David Fairhurst. "Engaging a new generation of graduates." *Education + Training*, 50, no. 5 (2008): 366 – 378.

Somunoğlu, Sinem, Erhan Erdem, and Ümmühan Erdem. "A study on determining the perception of learning organisation applications by health sector workers." *Journal of medical systems* 36, no. 6 (2012): 3925-3931.

Strauss, William, and Neil Howe. *Generations: The History of America's Future, 1584 to 2069.* New York: William Morrow and Company, 1991.

Swenson, Cathy. "Next Generation Workforce." *Nursing Economics* 26, no. 9 (2008).

Tajfel, Henri, and John C. Turner. (Ed.). "The social identity theory of intergroup behavior." In S. Worchel and W. G. Austin (eds) Psychology of intergroup relations 2nd ed (1986): 7-24. Chicago Nelson-Hall.

Taylor, Jeannette. "Organizational influences, public service motivation and work outcomes: An Australian study." *International Public Management Journal* 11, no. 1 (2008): 67-88.

Terjesen, Siri, Susan Vinnicombe, and Cheryl Freeman. "Attracting generation Y Graduates: Organisational Attributes, Likelihood to Apply and Sex Differences." *Career Development International* 12, no. 6 (2007): 504-22.

Twenge, Jean M., and Stacy M. Campbell. "Generational Differences In Psychological Traits And Their Impact On The Workplace." *Journal of Managerial Psychology* 23, no. 8 (2008): 862-77.

Van Dick, Rolf, Michael W. Grojean, Oliver Christ, and Jan Wieseke. "Identity and the extra mile: Relationships between organizational identification and organizational citizenship behavior." *British Journal of Management, 17* (2006): 283-301

Wong, Melissa, Elliroma Gardiner, Whitney Lang, and Leah Coulon. "Generational Differences In Personality And Motivation: Do They

Exist And What Are The Implications For The Workplace?" *Journal of Managerial Psychology* 23 (2008): 878-90.

Wright, Patrick M., and Rebecca R. Kehoe. "Human Resource Practices And Organizational Commitment: A Deeper Examination." *Asia Pacific Journal of Human Resources* 46, no. 1 (2007): 6-20.

Yrle, Augusta C., Sandra J. Hartman, and Dinah M. Payne. "Generation X: Acceptance of Others and Teamwork Implications." *Team Performance Management: An International Journal Team Performance Management* 11, no. 5.6 (2005): 188-99.

Zangaro, George A. "Organizational Commitment: A Concept Analysis." *Nursing Forum* 36, no. 2 (2001): 14-21.

Further Readings

Adams, Ann, and Senga Bond. "Hospital nurses' job satisfaction, individual and organizational characteristics." *Journal of advanced nursing* 32, no. 3 (2000): 536-543.

Albert, Stuart, Blake E. Ashforth, and Jane E. Dutton. "Organizational Identity And Identification: Charting New Waters And Building New Bridges." *Academy of Management Review* 25, no. 1 (2000): 13-17.

Allen, Natalie. "Affective, Continuance, And Normative Commitment To The Organization: An Examination Of Construct Validity." *Journal of Vocational Behavior* 49, no. 3 (1996): 252-76. doi:10.10006/jvbe.1996.0043.

Allen, Natalie J., and John P. Meyer. "The Measurement and Antecedents of Affective, Continuance and Normative Commitment to the Organization." *Journal of Occupational Psychology* 63, no. 1 (1990): 1-18.

Allison, David B., and Bernard S. Gorman. "Some of Them Most Common Questions Asked of Statistical Consultants: Our Favorite Responses and Recommended Readings." *Journal of Group Psychotherapy, Psychodrama, and Sociometry* 46 (1993): 83-103.

Amos, Elizabeth A., and Bart L. Weathington. "An Analysis of the Relation Between Employee—Organization Value Congruence and Employee Attitudes." *The Journal of Psychology* 142, no. 6 (2008): 615-32.

Apostolidis, Beka M., and E. Carol Polifroni. "Nurse Work Satisfaction and Generational Differences." *JONA: The Journal of Nursing Administration* 36, no. 11 (2006): 506-09.

Asthana, Anushka. "Generation Y: They Don't Live for Work, They Work to Live." *The Observer* (2008). Accessed May 21, 2015. http://www.guardian.co.uk/money/2008/may/25/workandcareers.worklifebalance.

Benson, John, and Michelle Brown. "Generations At Work: Are There Differences And Do They Matter?" *The International Journal of Human Resource Management* 22, no. 9 (2011): 1843-865.

Blythe, Jennifer, Andrea Baumann, Isik U. Zeytinoglu, Margaret Denton, Noori Akhtar-Danesh, Sharon Davies, and Camille Kolotylo. "Nursing Generations in the Contemporary Workplace." *Public Personnel Management* 37, no. 2 (2008): 137-59. Accessed May 21, 2015. http://search.proquest.com/docview/215933963?accountid=14872.

Bracken, David W., and Dale S. Rose. "When does 360-degree Feedback create behavior change? And How would we know when it does?" *Journal of Business and Psychology* 26, no. 2 (2011).

Bridges, Andrew. "Meeting the Needs and Expectations of generation X and generation Y Employees." Strange Attractors Challenge Team Project Report. 2007. Accessed May 21, 2015.

Brunetto, Yvonne, Matthew Xerri, Art Shriberg, Rod Farr-Wharton, Kate Shacklock, Stefanie Newman, and Joy Dienger. "The Impact of Workplace Relationships on Engagement, Well-being, Commitment and Turnover for Nurses in Australia and the USA." *Journal of Advanced Nursing* 69, no. 12 (2013): 2786-799. doi:10.1111/jan.12165.

Bureau of Labor Statistics, U.S. Department of Labor, *Occupational Outlook Handbook, 2012-13 Edition*, Registered Nurses, Retrieved from http://www.bls.gov/ooh/healthcare/registered-nurses.htm.

Chew, Janet, and Christopher C.A. Chan. "Human Resource Practices, Organizational Commitment And Intention To Stay." *International Journal of Manpower* 29, no. 6 (2008): 503-22.

Cottingham, Stacy, Mary C. Dibartolo, Susan Battistoni, and Tina Brown. "Partners In Nursing:." *Nursing Education Perspectives* 32, no. 4 (2011): 250-55. doi:10.5480/1536-5026-32.4.250.

Creswell, John W. *Educational Research: Planning, Conducting, and Evaluating Quantitative and Qualitative Research.* 2nd ed. Upper Saddle River, N.J.: Pearson/Merrill Prentice Hall, 2004.

Creswell, John W., and John W. Creswell. *Qualitative Inquiry and Research Design: Choosing among Five Approaches.* Thousand Oaks: SAGE Publications, 2009.

Daniels, Frieda, Audrey Laporte, Louise Lemieux-Charles, Andrea Baumann, Kanecy Onate, and Raisa Deber. "The Importance of Employment Status in Determining Exit Rates From Nursing." *Nursing Economic$* 30, no. 4 (2012).

Deal, Jennifer J. *Retiring the Generation Gap: How Employees Young and Old Can Find Common Ground.* San Francisco, CA: Wiley, 2007.

Disch, Joanne, Sandra Edwardson, and Jehad Adwan. "Nursing Faculty Satisfaction with Individual, Institutional, and Leadership Factors." *Journal of Professional Nursing* 20, no. 5 (2004): 323-32.

Dobransky-Fasiska, D. G. "A discriminate analysis of entrepreneurial personality characteristics for each of three generational cohorts: The silent generation, the baby boomers and generation X." Doctoral diss., 2002, ProQuest (765190511).

Dorgham, Shereen Ragab. "Relationship between Organization Work Climate and Staff Nurses Organization Commitment." *Nature and Science* 15, no. 5 (2012): 80-91.

El-Jardali, Fadi, Mirvat Merhi, Diana Jamal, Nuhad Dumit, and Gladys Mouro. "Assessment of Nurse Retention Challenges and Strategies in Lebanese Hospitals: The Perspective of Nursing Directors." *Journal of Nursing Management* 17, no. 4 (2009): 453-62. doi:10.1111/j.1365-2834.2009.00972.x.

Erdem, R. (2007). Örgüt kültürü tipleri ile örgütsel bağlılık arasındaki ilişki: Elazığ il merkezindeki hastaneler üzerinde bir çalışma (the relationship between organizational culture types and organişzational commitment: A study on hospitals at Elazığ central municipality). Eskişehir Osmangazi Üniversitesi İİBF Dergisi, 2(2), 63-79.

Farr-Wharton, Rod, Yvonne Brunetto, and Kate Shacklock. "The Impact of Intuition and Supervisor-nurse Relationships on Empowerment and Affective Commitment by Generation." *Journal of Advanced Nursing* 68, no. 6 (2012): 1391-401. doi:10.1111/j.1365-2648.2011.05852.x.

Gambino, Kathleen M. "Motivation for Entry, Occupational Commitment and Intent to Remain: A Survey regarding Registered Nurse Retention." *Journal of Advanced Nursing* 66, no. 11 (2010): 2532-541. doi:10.1111/j.1365-2648.2010.05426.x.

Gelade, Garry A., Paul Dobson, and Patrick Gilbert. "National Differences In Organizational Commitment: Effect of Economy, Product of Personality, or Consequence of Culture?" *Journal of Cross-Cultural Psychology* 37 (2006): 542-56.

George, Darren, and Paul Mallery. *SPSS for Windows Step by Step: A Simple Guide and Reference, 15.0 Update.* 8th ed. Boston: Pearson/A and B, 2008.

Goulet, Laurel R., and Margaret L. Frank. "Organizational Commitment across Three Sectors: Public, Non-profit, and For-profit." *Public Personnel Management* 31, no. 2 (2002): 201-210.

Gravetter, Frederick J., and Larry B. Wallnau. *Statistics for the Behavioral Sciences.* 8th ed. Belmont, CA: Wadsworth, 2009.

Gök, Ayşen Uğur, and Gülseren Kocaman. "Reasons for Leaving Nursing: A Study among Turkish Nurses." *Contemporary Nurse* 39, no. 1 (2011): 65-74.

Harris, Sandra M. "Development of the Perceptions of Mentoring Relationships Survey (PMRS): A Mixed Methods Approach." *International Journal of Multiple Research Approaches* 7, no. 1 (2013): 2405-2439.

Hertel, Bradley R. "Minimizing Error Variance Introduced By Missing Data Routines in Survey Analysis." *Sociological Methods Research,* (1976): 459-474. doi:10.1177/00491241760040040.

Hoffman, Helen. "A Nurse Retention Program." *Nursing Economic$* 7, no. 2 (1989): 94-108.

Hogan, Pamela, Lorna Moxham, and Trudy Dwyer. "Human Resource Management Strategies for the Retention of Nurses in Acute Care Settings in Hospitals in Australia." *Contemporary Nurse* 24, no. 2 (2007): 189-199.

Howell, David C. *Fundamental Statistics for the Behavioral Sciences.* 5th ed. Belmont: Brooks-Cole, 2004.

Johnson, Russell E., and Liu-Qin Yang. "Commitment and motivation at work: The relevance of employee identity and regulatory focus." *Academy of Management Review* 35, no. 2 (2010): 226-245.

Jones, April. "Generational cohort differences among nurses types of organizational commitment in Alabama." 2014. ProQuest (3645920).

Kaplan, Robert M., and Dennis P. Saccuzzo. *Psychological Testing: Principles, Applications, and Issues.* 6th ed. Belmont, CA: Wadsworth-Thompson, 2005.

Kooker, Barbara Molina, and Cynthia Kamikawa. "Successful Strategies to Improve RN Retention and Patient Outcomes in a Large Medical Centre in Hawaii." *Journal of Clinical Nursing* 20, no. 1/2 (2011): 34-39. doi:10.1111/j.1365-2702.2010.03476.x.

Lamm, Eric, and Michael D. Meeks. "Workplace fun: the moderating effects of generational differences." *Employee relations* 31, no. 6 (2009): 613-631.

Leedy, Paul D., and Jeanne Ellis Ormrod. *Practical Research: Planning and Design.* 8th ed. Upper Saddle River, N.J.: Prentice Hall, 2001.

Macky, Keith, Dianne Gardner, and Stewart Forsyth. "Generational Differences At Work: Introduction And Overview." *Journal of Managerial Psychology* 23, no. 8 (2008): 857-861. doi:10.1108/02683940810904358.

Mayer, Roger C., and F. David Schoorman. "Predicting Participation And Production Outcomes Through A Two-Dimensional Model Of Organizational Commitment." *Academy of Management Journal* 35, no. 3 (1992): 671-684.

McCreless, P. - The Anniston, S. "Alabama sees shortage of nurses, truck drivers." *AP Regional State Report – Alabama.*(2013)

McNeese-Smith, Donna, and Margaret Nazarey. "A Nursing Shortage: Building Organizational Commitment among Nurses / Practitioner Application." *Journal of Healthcare Management* 46, no. 3 (2001): 173-186.

Mertler, Craig A., and Rachel A. Vannatta. *Advanced and Multivariate Statistical Methods: Practical Application and Interpretation.* 3rd ed. Glendale, CA: Pyrczak, 2005.

Meyer, John. "Affective, Continuance, And Normative Commitment To The Organization: A Meta-analysis Of Antecedents, Correlates, And Consequences." *Journal of Vocational Behavior* 61, no. 1 (2002): 20-52.

Meyer, John P., Natalie J. Allen, and Catherine A. Smith. "Commitment to Organizations and Occupations: Extension and Test of a Three-component Conceptualization." *Journal of Applied Psychology* 78, no. 4 (1993): 538-551. doi:10.1037/0021-9010. 78.4.538.

Molloy, Geoffrey N. *SPSS Survival Manual a Step by Step Guide to Data Analysis Using SPSS.* 4th ed. Maidenhead: Open University Press/ McGraw-Hill, 2001.

Montana, Patrick J., and Francis Petit. "Motivating generation X and Y on the Job and Preparing Z." *Global Journal of Business Research* 2, no. 2 (2008): 139-148.

Morgan, Jennifer Craft, and Mary R. Lynn. "Satisfaction In Nursing In The Context Of Shortage." *Journal of Nursing Management* 17, no. 3 (2009): 401-10. doi:10.1111/j.1365-2834.2007.00842.x.

Mosadeghrad, Ali Mohammad, Ewan Ferlie, and Duska Rosenberg. "A Study of the Relationship between Job Satisfaction, Organizational Commitment and Turnover Intention among Hospital Employees." *Health Services Management Research* 21, no. 4 (2008): 211-27. doi:10.1258/hsmr.2007.007015.

Neutens, James J., and Laurna Rubinson. *Research Techniques for the Health Sciences*. 4th ed. San Francisco: B. Cummings, 2010.

Norman, Steven M., James B. Avey, James L. Nimnicht, and Nancy Graber Pigeon. "The interactive effects of psychological capital and organizational identity on employee citizenship and deviance behaviors." *Journal of Leadership & Organizational Studies* (2010).

Norman, Steve, Brett Luthans, and Kyle Luthans. "The proposed contagion effect of hopeful leaders on the resiliency of employees and organizations."*Journal of Leadership & Organizational Studies* 12, no. 2 (2005): 55-64.

Norman, Paul, and Celia Bonnett. "Managers' Intentions to be Assessed for Vocational Qualifications: An Application of the Theory of Planned Behavior." *Social Behavior and Personality: an international journal* 23, no. 1 (1995): 59-67.

O'donnell, Deanna, Patricia M Livingston, and Timothy Bartram. "Human Resource Management Activities on the Front Line: A Nursing Perspective." *Contemporary Nurse*, 2012, 198-205.

"Occupational Outlook Handbook." U.S. Bureau of Labor Statistics. Accessed May 21, 2015.

Onwuegbuzie, Anthony J., and Larry G. Daniel. "Typology of Analytical and Interpretational Errors in Quantitative and Qualitative Educational Research." *Current Issues in Education* 6, no. 2 (2003).

Pallant, Julie. *SPSS Survival Manual a Step by Step Guide to Data Analysis Using SPSS.* 4th ed. Berkshire, England: Open University Press/ McGraw-Hill, 2007.

Palumbo, Mary Val, Barbara McIntosh, Betty Rambur, and Shelly Naud. "Retaining an Aging Nurse Workforce: Perceptions of Human Resource Practices." *Nursing Economic$* 27, no. 4 (2009): 221-232.

Papinczak, Tracey. "Perceptions of Job Satisfaction Relating to Affective Organisation Commitment." *Medical Education* 46, no. 10 (2012): 953-62. doi:10.1111/j.1365-2923.2012.04314.x.

Parry, Emma, and Peter Urwin. "Generational Differences In Work Values: A Review Of Theory And Evidence." *International Journal of Management Reviews*, 2010. doi:10.1111/j.1468-2370.2010.00285x.

Pilcher, Jane. "Mannheim's Sociology of Generations: An Undervalued Legacy." *The British Journal of Sociology* 45, no. 3 (1994): 481.

Randall, Donna M. "Commitment and the Organization: The Organization Man Revisited." *Academy of Management Review* 12, no. 3 (1987): 460.

Randall, Donna M. "The Consequences of Organizational Commitment: Methodological Investigation." *Journal of Organizational Behavior* 11, no. 5 (1990): 361-78.

Ray, Tiffany "Alabama hospitals scramble to recruit, retain qualified nurses with pay, perks." *Knight Ridder Tribune Business News.* August 29, 2004. http://search.proquest.com/docview/463825762?accoun tid=14872

Rea, Louis M., and Richard A. Parker. *Designing and Conducting Survey Research. A Comprehensive Guide.* San Francisco, CA: Jossey-Bass, 2005.

Seidl, Wolfgang. "Meeting demands of generation Y should be HR's target." *Personnel Today* (2008). Retrieved from http://www.person-neltoday.com/articles/2008/04/03/45231/meeting-demands-of-generation-y-should-be-hrs-target.html.

Slogan Center of Aging and Work. *Age and the Meaning of Work* (2008). Retrieved from www.bc.edu/research/agingandwork/projects/meaning ofwork.html.

Somers, Mark John. "Patterns of Attachment to Organizations: Commitment Profiles and Work Outcomes." *Journal of Occupational and Organizational Psychology* 83, no. 2 (2010): 443-53. doi:10.1348/096317909X424060.

Spetz, Joanne, and Ruth Given. "The Future Of The Nurse Shortage: Will Wage Increases Close The Gap?" *Health Affairs* 22, no. 6 (2003): 199-206.

SPSS. *Behaviour Change* 18.1: 58-58. Retrieved from http://search.pro-quest.com/docview/219355175?accountid=14872 personality and motivation: Do they exist and what are the implications for the work-place?" *Journal of Managerial Psychology* 23 (2008): 878-890.

Stevens, James. *Applied Multivariate Statistics for the Social Sciences.* 5th ed. New York, NY: Routledge, 2009.

Taylor, M. Susan, Giuseppe Audia, and Anil K. Gupta. "The effect of lengthening job tenure on managers' organizational commitment and turnover."*Organization Science* 7, no. 6 (1996): 632-648.

Taylor, Sully, Orly Levy, Nakiye A. Boyacigiller, and Schon Beechler. "Employee commitment in MNCs: Impacts of organizational culture, HRM and top management orientations." *The International Journal of Human Resource Management,* 19, no. 4 (2008): 501-527.

Tourangeau, Ann E., Greta Cummings, Lisa A. Cranley, Era Mae Ferron, and Sarah Harvey. "Determinants of Hospital Nurse Intention to Remain Employed: Broadening Our Understanding." *Journal of Advanced Nursing* 66, no. 1 (2009): 22-32. doi:10.1111/j.1365-2648.2009.05190.x.

Tourangeau, Ann E., Heather Thomson, Greta Cummings, and Lisa A. Cranley. "Generation-specific Incentives and Disincentives for Nurses to Remain Employed in Acute Care Hospitals." *Journal of Nursing Management* 21, no. 3 (2013): 473-82. doi:10.1111/j.1365-2834.2012.01424.x.

Trochim, William M. K. *Research Methods Knowledge Base.* 2nd ed. Cincinnati, OH: Atomic Dog Pub., 2001.

Veurink, Shannon A., and Ronald Fischer. "A Refocus on Foci: A Multidimensional and Multi-foci Examination of Commitment in Work Contexts." *New Zealand Journal Of Psychology* 40, no. 3 (2001): 160-167.

Wallis, Allan, and Kathy I. Kennedy. "Leadership Training to Improve Nurse Retention." *Journal of Nursing Management* 21, no. 4 (2013): 624-632. doi:10.1111/j.1365-2834.2012.01443.x.

Westhuis, David, and Bruce A. Thyer. "Development And Validation Of The Clinical Anxiety Scale: A Rapid Assessment Instrument For Empirical Practice." *Educational and Psychological Measurement* 49 (1989): 153-63. doi:10.1177/0013164489491016.

Wieck, K. Lynn, Jean Dols, and Peggy Landrum. "Retention Priorities For The Intergenerational Nurse Workforce." *Nursing Forum* 45, no. 1 (2010): 7-17.

Wilkinson, Leland. "Statistical Methods In Psychology Journals: Guidelines And Explanations." *American Psychologist* 54, no. 8 (1999): 594-604.

Yaget, K. "A Study on Measuring the Levels of Organizational Commitment of the Hotel Workers by Means of Approach by Meyer-Allen Organization Commitment Model." *Journal of Institute of Social Science* 9, no. 3 (2007): 114-129.

Yousef, Darwish A. "Organizational Commitment and Job Satisfaction as Prectictors of Attitudes toward Organizational Change in a Non-Western Setting." *Personnel Review* 29, no. 5 (2000): 567-592.

Yücel, Ilhami. "Examining the Relationships among Job Satisfaction, Organizational Commitment, and Turnover Intention: An Empirical Study." *International Journal of Business and Management* 7, no. 20 (2012). doi:10.5539/ijbm.v7n20p44.

Zimmerer, Tatiana Ekaterina. "Generation perceptions of servant leadership: A mixed method study." Doctoral Dissertation, 2013. ProQuest.

Index

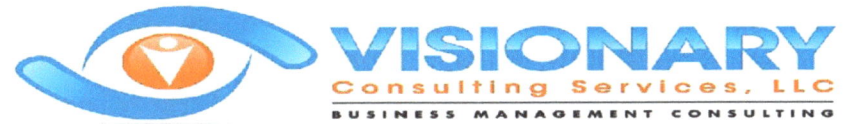

Go Further with VCS, LLC.

Website: www.vcsllc.co
Email: draljones@vcsllc.co   Phone: 334.277.8937

VCS, LLC is a business management consultant firm dedicated to providing dynamic management solutions geared toward the 21st Century and beyond. Our comprehensive suite of consulting services are custom designed by our experts to provide for maximum benefits and the flexibility our customers demand. We offer web-based, on-demand training and services as well as on-site organizational development courses that fit the needs of any business, regardless of size or strategic goals. Our experts utilize the latest research-based best practices to provide comprehensive, dynamic and effective development programs. For a full list of services and opportunities for your business or organization, visit our website at www.vcsllc.co today, and learn what Visionary Consulting Services can do for you. The company is headquartered in Montgomery, AL, U.S.